HANDBOOK
OF
OVARIAN CANCER
1ST EDITION

Acknowledgements

I would like to acknowledge my teacher Dr. Ramlingappa C A, Head of Department, OBG, Karnataka Institute of Medical Sciences; for his encouragement & support during my post graduation.

In addition a thank you to my present unit chief Dr. Vinita Singh, Tata Main Hospital; for her continuous support and guidance during my reading work and writing.

Finally, I would like to thank my bird, my parents for their unconditional love and support .

Preface

Worldwide, 204,449 new cases of ovarian cancer are diagnosed each year, with an estimated 124,860 disease-related deaths. There are notable differences in ovarian cancer incidence across the world. In Europe, in 2012, there were 65,538 cases with a mortality rate of 42,704 women. The American Cancer Society's estimates for ovarian cancer in the USA for 2013 are: about 22,240 women will receive a new diagnosis of ovarian cancer and about 14,230 women will die from the disease. The ovarian cancer statistics for incidence indicates it is highest in the USA and Northern Europe and lowest in Africa and Asia. Ovarian cancer is the ninth most common cancer among women, excluding nonmelanoma skin cancers. It ranks fifth in cancer deaths among women. It accounts for about 3 % of all cancers in women. A woman's risk of getting ovarian cancer during her lifetime is about 1 in 72. Her lifetime chance of dying from ovarian cancer is about 1 in 100. Incidence rates of ovarian cancer increase with age, becoming more prevalent in the eighth decade of life. Patients are typically diagnosed when the disease has metastasized (stage III or IV) which has an overall survival rate between 5 and 25 %.

Five-year survival in ovarian cancer has doubled over the past 30 years, increasing from approximately 25 % to 50 %. This is a result of developments in diagnosis and more efficient management. Clearly, there is more room to increase this rate to a higher number. This could be achieved by developing novel tests for early detection and diagnosis and innovative medical therapy and surgical techniques. The ideal approach to women with ovarian cancer is a multidisciplinary one, with many professionals contributing to the excellent care and outcome that we wish to see for those individuals we are privileged to look after.

This book is intended for all postgraduates of obstetrics and gynecology & clinicians caring for women with ovarian cancer, including attending surgeons and physicians, fellows, and residents in the disciplines of gynecologic oncology, surgical oncology, medical oncology, and primary care as an useful adjunct to getting current information on diagnosis and management of ovarian cancer.

Prashant Pujara.
Tata Main Hostpital, Jamshedpur

CONTENETS

EPITHELIAL OVARIAN CARCINOMA

GERM CELL MALIGNANCIES

1. INTRODUCTION/EPIDEMIOLOGY
2. ORIGIN
3. CLASSIFICATION
4. ETIOLOGY & RISK FACTORS
5. DYSGERMINOMA
6. IMMATURE TERATOMAS
7. ENDODERMAL SINUS TUMORS
8. EMBRYONAL CARCINOMA
9. CHORIOCARCINOMA OF THE OVARY
10. POLYEMBRYOMA
11. MIXED GERM CELL TUMORS
12. MANAGEMENT
    - Primary treatment
    - Follow-up/monitoring
13. MANAGEMENT OF RECURRENT DISEASE
14. MANAGEMENT DURING PREGNANCY
15. LATE EFFECTS OF TREATMENT OF MALIGNANT GERM CELL TUMORS
    - Gonadal function
    - Secondary malignancies

GERM CELL MALIGNANCIES

1. INTRODUCTION/EPIDEMIOLOGY
2. ORIGIN
3. CLASSIFICATION
4. GRANULOSA-STROMAL CELL TUMORS
5. SERTOLI-LEYDIG TUMORS
6. MANAGEMENT
    - Primary treatment
    - Follow-up/monitoring
7. MANAGEMENT OF RECURRENT DISEASE

UNCOMMON OVARIAN CANCERS

METASTATIC TUMORS

MISCELLANEOUS

1. ROLE OF LAPAROSCOPY IN THE MANAGEMENT OF OVARIAN CANCER
2. FERTILITY SPARING SURGERY (FSS)
3. INTESTINAL OBSTRUCTION

OVARIAN CANCER

INTRODUCTION/EPIDEMIOLOGY

- 20% of ovarian neoplasms are malignant. **90% of malignant ovarian tumors in adults are of epithelial origin** f/b sex cord stromal tumors (6%) and germ-cell tumors (3%).

Ovarian cancer is the leading cause of death from gynecologic malignancies in the US & UK (T15) and is the US's fifth most common cause of cancer mortality in women. (N15)

- **The LR** for ovarian cancer in American women without a family history of the disease **is 1 in 70 (1.4%) & 2% in UK.**

- Highest → Sweden and US (Caucasian > African American > Native American).
- Lowest → Japan.
- **India → 4.6/1,00,000.**

CLINICAL PRESENTATION

SYMPTOMS

EARLY STAGE	ADVANCED STAGE	4 TARGET SYMPTOMS
Silent disease, nonspecific symptoms like, - Abdominal bloating or pain, - Indigestion (flatulence), - Loss of appetite, - If a pelvic mass is compressing the bladder or rectum, urinary frequency or constipation, - Irregular menses, - Lower abdominal distention, pressure or pain (dyspareunia) [rare], - Acute pain due to rupture or torsion (rare) [D/D acute appendicitis].	- Abdominal swelling which may be rapid, - Dull abdominal pain, - Respiratory distress (ascites/pleural effusion), - Bloating, constipation, anorexia, early satiety, - Fatigue, - Weight loss. - Endometrial hyperplasia and AUB is absent except in functioning ovarian tumor (excess estrogen production from an ovarian stromal tumor) & can cause irregular, heavy menses or postmenopausal bleeding - **Vaginal bleeding** is seen with metastatic involvement of the uterus - Postmenopausal bleeding	- Abdominal pain (MC), - Abdominal swelling, - GI symptoms, & - Pelvic pain. ↓ High index of suspicion + pelvic ultrasound + CA-125. ↓ May lead to earlier diagnosis.

GERM CELL MALIGNANCIES
- In contrast to slow-growing EOCs, germ cell malignancies **grow rapidly** and characterized **by subacute pelvic pain (capsular distention, hemorrhage, or necrosis).**

- Young patients may misinterpret the **early symptoms as those of** pregnancy (delay in the diagnosis).

SIGNS

G/E:

- Cachexia & pallor.
- Icterus in late cases.

- Shortness of breath.
- Left supraclavicular lymph nodes (Virchow's) may be enlarged.
- Oedema of leg or vulva is characteristic of malignant tumor.
- Signs of virilization (**oligomenorrhea followed by amenorrhea, breast atrophy, acne, hirsutism, clitoromegaly, deepening of the voice, and a receding hairline**) & precocious puberty (steroid producing ovarian tumors).

S/E:

- A malignant **pleural effusion on the right side** from metastasis is usually associated with dullness to percussion and on auscultation ↓sed breath sounds.

P/A:

- Liver may be enlarged, firm & nodular.
- Ascites.
- A pelvic mass (**most important sign**) is felt in the hypogastrium; too often it may be bilateral. It has got following features:
  - Feel- Solid or heterogenous.
  - Mobility- Mobile or restricted.
  - Tenderness- Usually present.
  - Surfaces- Irregular.
  - Margins- Well-defined but the lower pole is usually not reached.
  - Percussion- Usually dull over the tumor; may be resonant due to overlying intestinal adhesions.
- Palpable adnexal mass in premenarcheal patient (?germ cell tumors) requires EUA.
- Palpation of both groins to rule out **inguinal lymphadenopathy** secondary to metastatic disease.

P/V:

- Any palpable pelvic mass in 1 year postmenopausal women should be considered potentially malignant (ovaries should be atrophic), referred to as the **postmenopausal palpable ovary syndrome**. This concept has been challenged, because only about 3% of palpable masses measuring <5 cm in postmenopausal women are malignant.
- The uterus is separated from the mass felt per abdomen. A groove or cleft between ovarian tumor and uterus is called **"Hangoranis sign"**.
- Nodules may be felt through the posterior fornix. If it is more than 1 cm, the diagnosis of malignancy is almost certain.

EARLY DETECTION/SCREENING

- **For screening to be effective**, a disease should...
(a) Be a major cause of mortality,
(b) Have a reasonably high prevalence in the screened population,
(c) Have a preclinical phase detectable by the screening test, and
(d) Be amenable to therapy, such that the survival rate of patients with early-stage disease is significantly higher than that of patients with advanced disease.

- **Characteristics of an optimal screening test** include...
(a) High sensitivity & specificity,
(b) High PPV & NPV.

- The test should be easy to perform, time efficient, and well accepted by patients.

- **An effective screening test** should...
(a) Decrease stage at detection,
(b) Decrease case-specific mortality, and
(c) Cause a statistically significant reduction in site-specific cancer mortality in the screened population.

- Finally, the screening test should be cost-effective, such that its use would reduce the overall cost of health care in the screened population.

- Routine yearly pelvic examination has not been shown to increase the diagnosis of early-stage ovarian cancer. Pelvic examination is inaccurate in assessing ovarian size, particularly in postmenopausal or overweight women.

1) OVARIAN CANCER SYMPTOM INDEX

- Carry out tests in primary care if a woman (especially if 50 or over) reports having any of the following symptoms on a persistent or frequent basis particularly >12 days/month...
- Persistent abdominal distension ('bloating')
- Feeling full (early satiety) and/or loss of appetite
- Pelvic or abdominal pain
- Increased urinary urgency and/or frequency. (R11)

Especially if these symptoms are new (<1 year). (N15)

- Carry out tests for ovarian cancer in any woman of 50 or over who has experienced symptoms within the last 12 months that suggest IBS, because IBS rarely presents for the first time in women of this age. (R11)

- Measure serum CA125 in primary care in women with symptoms that suggest ovarian cancer.
- If ≥35 IU/ml, arrange an ultrasound scan of the abdomen and pelvis. Calculate a RMI I score after ultrasound; and refer all with an RMI I score of ≥250 to a specialist multidisciplinary team.
- If normal serum CA125 (<35 IU/ml), or CA125 of 35 IU/ml or greater but a normal ultrasound:
    - Assess carefully for other clinical causes of her symptoms and investigate if appropriate

       o   If no other clinical cause is apparent, advise her to return to her GP if her symptoms become more frequent and/or persistent. (R11)

2) TVS

- Using **5.0-mHz vaginal transducer,** complete screening takes **5-10 minutes** and is **painless.**

- Each ovary is measured in three dimensions, and **ovarian volume is calculated using the prolate ellipsoid formula** (L × H × W × 0.523)...
- >20 cm^3 **in premenopausal women** or
- >10 cm^3 **in postmenopausal women** is defined as abnormal.
- Any **solid or papillary projection from the tumor wall** is considered abnormal.

Pros: The sensitivity of TVS is 85%, and the specificity is 98.8%.

Cons: However, the PPV of TVS screening in detecting ovarian cancer is only 13.8%. Additional tests that can increase the PPV of TVS must be developed. Adjuvant method capable of increasing the PPV of TVS screening is morphology indexing.

3) CA 125

- CA-125 is an antigenic determinant on a HMW glycoprotein recognized by a monoclonal antibody, OC-125.

- It can be used **independently or in conjunction with sonographic findings** in screening high risk population or to differentiate benign from malignant ovarian tumors.

- CA-125 is expressed by EOCs and is present in highest concentrations on the tumor cell surface.

- **Serum levels are elevated (>35 µ/mL) in...**
- 80% of patients with advanced ovarian cancer.
- 25-50% of stage I ovarian cancers.
- Benign ovarian conditions, such as **endometriomas, inflammatory disease of the ovaries, and serous cystadenomas.**
- Nongynecologic cancers of the **pancreas, breast, colon, and lung.**

- Because many of the benign conditions producing elevated serum marker levels occur in younger women, the specificity of serum CA-125 is highest in postmenopausal women.

Pros: Single serum CA-125 has a specificity of 98.5%.

Cons: Single serum CA-125 has a sensitivity of 58% and a PPV of 2%. When serum CA-125 was used as the initial screening method, <u>early-stage cancers were missed,</u> and <u>stage at detection was not decreased appreciably.</u>

- **Rising trend in serum CA-125 levels over time (2-4 weeks) is more predictive of ovarian cancer than a single elevated marker (can be present in benign condition) determination.** The specificity of CA125 is improved when the test is combined with TVS or TAS or when the CA125 levels are followed over time.

4) RISK OF OVARIAN CANCER ALGORITHM (ROCA):

- ROCA was originally developed using data from prospective screening trials for postmenopausal women that included more than 22,000 women in the United Kingdom and more than 5000 women in Sweden. Statistical analysis of these data indicated most women without ovarian cancer had a flat CA125 profile, namely, a baseline level individual to each woman around which her CA125 levels fluctuated. In contrast, women with incident cases of ovarian cancer had a baseline level followed by a sharp increase in CA125 values significantly above her baseline, called a change-point CA125 profile, which could not be explained by background CA125 fluctuations. These thousands of profiles form the basis for the ROCA calculation that determines a woman's risk of having ovarian cancer at that time

- ROCA compares the profile of CA125 results in a woman, to other known CA125 profiles from healthy women as well as those who have developed ovarian cancer.

CATEGORIES	ROCA RISK SCORE	RECOMMENDATION
Normal risk	<1 in 2000	Repeat CA-125 in 1 year
Intermedicate risk	1 in 2000 to 1 in 500	Repeat CA-125 in 3 months
Elevated risk	>1 in 500	TVS & referral to gynecologic oncologist

- ROCA measures the relative closeness of the woman's longitudinal CA125 pattern to the change-point profile in ovarian cancer cases from previous trials compared with the flat profiles seen in all other women without ovarian cancer in previous trial.

- No enough evidence to support this screening for women at low risk. ROCA may be useful for women at high risk (with BRCA mutations). (N15)

5) OTHER BIOMARKERS

- Another new approach is the measurement of plasma DNA levels and allelic imbalance by a technique known as **digital single nucleotide polymorphism (SNP) analysis.**

- The Society of Gynecologic Oncology (SGO), the FDA, and the Mayo Clinic have stated that the **OVA1 test** (using 5 biomarkers transthyretin, apolipoprotein A1, transferrin, beta-2 microglobulin, and CA-125) should not be used as a screening tool to detect ovarian cancer. (N15)

- NCCN believes that the **OvaSure screening test** (using 6 biomarkers leptin, prolactin, osteopontin, insulin-like growth factor II, macrophage inhibitory factor, and CA-125) should not be used to detect ovarian cancer. (N15)

CONCLUSION

- Combine **TVS with serum markers** in an algorithm improves the sensitivity, specificity, and PPV of screening.

- Currently available screening techniques are not sensitive or specific enough to recommend routine screening for general population. (N15) Screening of high-risk women (e.g., those with BRCA mutations, those with a family history) using CA-125 monitoring and TVS should be individualized. However prospective validation of these tests remains elusive.

An ongoing trial is assessing screening (**UK Collaborative Trial of Ovarian Cancer Screening [UKCTOCS]**) using multimodality screening with ultrasound and CA-125 versus either ultrasound alone or no screening. Preliminary results suggest that multimodality screening is more effective at detecting early-stage cancer.
However, a large randomized trial in more than 78,000 women (**the Prostate, Lung, Colorectal, and Ovarian [PLCO] Cancer trial**) in the US found that screening with TVS and CA-125 did not decrease mortality from ovarian cancer. In addition, false-positive results led to serious complications in some women (n = 163) in the PLCO trial.
Another study—comparing 1) CA-125 alone; 2) ultrasound with CA-125; or 3) ultrasound alone—found that CA-125 did not increase the detection of cancer over ultrasound alone and that ultrasound was superior to CA-125 alone.

ASSESSMENT OF RISK OF MALIGNANCY

1) CHARACTERISTICS OF MALIGNANCY

- Bilaterality,
- Solid composition,
- Fixation in the pelvis on bimanual examination, and
- Increased size (>10 cm diameter). **Extremely large ovarian tumors are often benign mucinous or serous cystadenomas.**
- **Consistency, contour & mobility of the lesion...**
    For the premenopausal patient...

<u>Mobile, mostly cystic, unilateral, and of regular contour adnexal mass</u>

No more than 2 months of observation during which hormonal suppression with OCP is given

Remain stable or regress → not neoplastic
Not regress or if increases in size or complexity → neoplastic → remove surgically

<u>Relatively fixed, predominantly solid, large, bilateral, and irregularly shaped</u>

Clinically suspicious

Laparotomy

2) ULTRASOUND

- TVS have better resolution than TAS for adnexal neoplasms. **Ultrasonographic signs of malignancy** include...
    - An adnexal pelvic mass with **areas of complexity, such as irregular borders, multiple echogenic patterns within the mass and dense multiple irregular septae.**
    - **Bilateral tumors,** although the individual characteristics of the lesions are of greater significance.

A. SIZE OF THE LESION:

- ≥2 cm adnexal mass in premenarcheal girl usually require exploration (N12),

- In postmenarcheal or premenopausal women... (N12)
    - ≤8 cm of predominantly cystic mass requires observation or OCP for 2 menstrual cycles,

- >8-10 cm of **complex cystic mass** can be neoplastic, unless the patient has been taking clomiphene citrate or other agents to induce ovulation

RCOG says (2011)

- <5 cm simple ovarian cysts do not require follow-up as these cysts are very likely to be physiological and almost always resolve within 3 menstrual cycles.
- 5-7 cm of simple ovarian cysts should have yearly ultrasound follow-up and
- >7 cm of simple cysts should be considered for either MRI or surgical intervention.

The use of the combined OCP does not promote the resolution of functional ovarian cysts

- In postmenopausal women... (N12)

- **Unilocular cysts measuring 8-10 cm or less (RCOG ≤5 cm) and normal serial CA125 levels, conservative management is acceptable,** and this may decrease the number of surgical interventions. Conservative management should entail repeat ultrasound scans and serum CA125 measurement every four months for one year. (R10)
- Complex adnexal masses of any size require laparotomy (bilateral oophorectomy should be done, cystectomy never).

[Ovarian cyst: 'a fluid-containing structure more than 30 mm in diameter'] [R11]

B. TUMOR MORPHOLOGY INDEX:

- Many morphology index are suggested to predict malignant potential of suspected ovarian mass. Out of them one of the most commonly used is DePriest ultrasound morphology index...

- The ultrasound morphology index is a cost-effective adjuvant method that significantly increases the specificity and positive predictive value of TVS and is based on the following...

- Tumour volume (<10 cm^3, 10 to 50 cm^3, >50 to 200 cm^3, >200 cm^3)

MORPHOLOGY INDEX

	OVARIAN VOLUME	WALL STRUCTURE	SEPTAE STRUCTURE
0	< 10 cm^3		
1	10-50 cm^3		
2	> 50-200 cm^3		
3	> 200-500 cm^3		
4	> 500 cm^3		

- Cyst wall structure and wall thickness (smooth <3 mm, smooth >3 mm, papillary <3 mm, papillary >3 mm)
- Septal structure (no septa, thin septa <3 mm, thick septa 3 to 10 mm, solid area >10 mm).

- A point scale (0 to 4) was developed within each category, with the total points per evaluation varying from 0 to 12.

- An ultrasound morphology index score <5 in a pre-menopausal woman is in keeping with a benign aetiology.
- In post-menopausal patients, a morphology index score ≥5 has a positive predictive value for malignancy of 0.45.

- Ovarian malignancies are more likely to have thickened wall structure and a total volume in excess of 10 cm^3.

- **Morphologic complexity and tumor volume (prolate ellipsoid formula)** $\propto$ **the risk of malignancy.**

3) CA 125

- It can be used **independently or in conjunction with sonographic findings** to differentiate benign from malignant ovarian tumors.

- Serum CA-125 **value >35 μ/mL is designated as abnormal.** Using this criterion, an elevated serum CA-125 in a postmenopausal woman with a sonographically confirmed ovarian tumor has a PPV for malignancy of 80% and sensitivity and specificity are also highest.

- **Serial CA 125 levels at 2- to 4-week intervals in a sonographically confirmed ovarian tumor may be more effective** than a single threshold value in distinguishing benign from malignant ovarian tumors.

- Serum CA125 levels...
- For a **postmenopausal patient** with **an adnexal mass** and a very **high serum CA125 level (>200 U/mL), there is a 96% PPV for malignancy.**
- For **premenopausal patients,** however, the **specificity of the test is low** because the **CA125 level tends to be elevated in common benign conditions.**

4) COLOR FLOW DOPPLER

- Tumor angiogenesis in neoplasia increases the number and tortuosity of vessels, which lack muscular intima and generally have low impedance to flow, in compare with normal ovarian tissue.

- A **PI of <1.0 and an RI of <0.4** are indicative of **low impedance to flow and a high risk of malignancy.**

- The overlap in values is such that preoperative color Doppler cannot be used as a reliable preoperative indicator of malignancy.

- Contrast-enhanced, 3-D power Doppler sonography can improve the visualization and diagnostic evaluation of tumor vascularity in complex adnexal masses. These are time-consuming and require sophisticated ultrasound equipment and sonographer skill. At present, Doppler flow studies are **used as adjunctive tests** in ovarian tumors suspected of being malignant on the basis of morphology indexing or serum marker patterns.

5) PROTEOMIC PROFILING OF SERUM

- Proteomic profiling of serum using mass spectroscopy [surface-enhanced laser desorption and ionization time of flight (SELDI-TOF)] also has been proposed as a method to differentiate benign from malignant ovarian tumors.

- A population of proteins can be profiled **according to the size and net electrical charge of the individual proteins.**

- The discriminating proteomic pattern formed by a subset of proteins is defined by peak amplitude at key mass/charge positions along the spectrum.

- These initial results have proven difficult to reproduce, and it is concluded that further work needs to be done.

6) RISK OF OVARIAN MALIGNANCY ALGORITHM

- **Serum HE4 and CA-125** along with an algorithm **(Risk of Ovarian Malignancy Algorithm [ROMA])** may be useful for determining whether a pelvic mass is malignant or benign. The FDA has approved HE4 and CA-125 for estimating the risk for ovarian cancer in women with a pelvic mass. Currently, NCCN does not recommend the use of these biomarkers for determining the status of an undiagnosed pelvic mass. (N15)

7) COMBINED MODALITIES

A. RISK OF MALIGNANCY INDEX (RMI)

- The RMI was first described by Jacobs in 1990 and has since evolved into RMI II, RMI III and RMI IV. To date only RMI I and RMI II have been sufficiently validated.

Feature	RMI 1 Score	RMI 2 Score	RMI 3 Score	RMI 4 Score
YEAR	Jacobs et al. 1990	Tingulstad et al. 1996	Tingulstad et al. 1999	Yamamoto et al. 2009
Ultrasound features: - multilocular cyst - solid areas - bilateral lesions - ascites - intra-abdominal metastases	0= none 1= one abnormality 3= two or more abnormalities	0= none 1= one abnormality 4= two or more abnormalities	1= none or one abnormality 3= two or more abnormalities	1= none or one abnormality 4= two or more abnormalities
Premenopausal	1	1	1	1
Postmenopausal	3	4	3	4
CA125	U/ml	U/ml	U/ml	U/ml
Tumor size (S) single greatest diameter	-	-	-	<7cm= 1 ≥7 cm= 2
RMI = ultrasound score x menopausal score x CA125 level in U/ml.				RMI = U x M x S x CA-125

- RMI 2 score gives greater weight to the ultrasound findings and menopausal status than the RMI 1 score. RMI 2 score is more sensitive than the RMI 1 system with results of 74 to 80% at a specificity of 89 to 92% and positive predictive values around 80.
- According to RMI 2 women are divided into...
  - Low-risk RMI = <25 (40% of women; risk of cancer is <3%).
  - Moderate-risk RMI = 25 to 250 (30% of women; risk of cancer is 20%).
  - High-risk RMI = >250 (30% of women; risk of cancer is 75%).

B. IOTA CLASSIFICATION

Risk of malignancy can be predicted preoperatively by various methods of IOTA (International Ovarian Tumor Analysis) group.

(1) IOTA classification using simple rules:

B-rules	M-rules
Unilocular cysts	Irregular solid tumour
Presence of solid components where the largest solid component <7 mm	Ascites
Presence of acoustic shadowing	At least four papillary structures
Smooth multilocular tumour with a largest diameter <100 mm	Irregular multilocular solid tumour with largest diameter ≥100 mm
No blood flow	Very strong blood flow

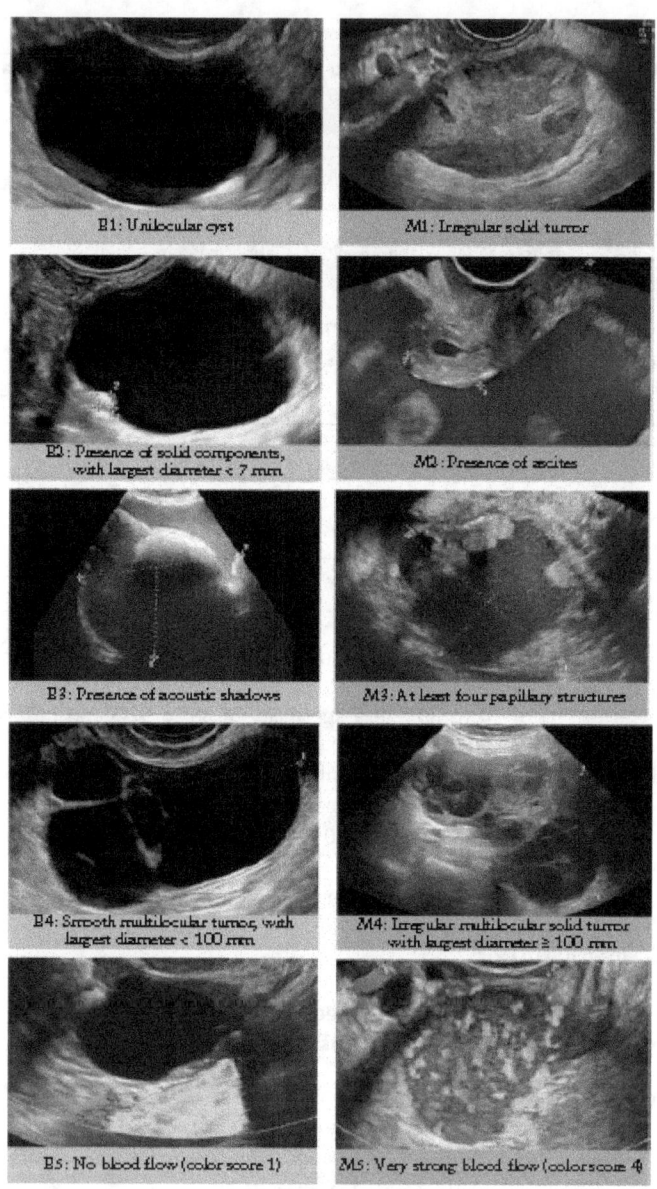

B1: Unilocular cyst

M1: Irregular solid tumor

B2: Presence of solid components, with largest diameter < 7 mm

M2: Presence of ascites

B3: Presence of acoustic shadows

M3: At least four papillary structures

B4: Smooth multilocular tumor, with largest diameter < 100 mm

M4: Irregular multilocular solid tumor with largest diameter ≥ 100 mm

B5: No blood flow (color score 1)

M5: Very strong blood flow (color score 4)

Rule 1: ≥1 M features + 0 B feature → Malignant.
Rule 2: ≥1 B features + 0 M feature → Benign.
Rule 3: If both M features and B features are present, or if no B or M features are present, result is inconclusive and second stage test is recommended.

(2) Using logistic regression models 1 & 2:

- The logistic regression model 1 is based on...
- The age of the patient (in years),
- The presence of ascites,
- The presence of blood flow within a papillary projection,
- The largest diameter of the solid component (in millimetres, but with no increase >50 mm),
- The presence of irregular internal cyst walls,
- The presence of acoustic shadows,
- Personal history of ovarian cancer,
- Current hormonal treatment,
- The largest diameter of the lesion (mm),
- Tenderness of the lesion during the examination,
- The presence of a purely solid tumour, and
- The colour score (1, 2, 3, or 4).

- The simpler logistic regression model (model 2) used only the first six variables. An estimated probability of malignancy above 0.10 by logistic regression model 1 or 2 classified the mass as malignant.

(3) IOTA-ADNEX model:

- ADNEX estimates the probability that an adnexal tumour is benign, borderline, stage I cancer, stage II-IV cancer, or secondary metastatic cancer

- The ADNEX uses nine predictors...
- 3 clinical variables, age, serum CA-125 level, and type of centre (oncology referral centre vs other), and
- 6 ultrasound variables, maximal diameter of lesion, proportion of solid tissue, more than 10 cyst locules, number of papillary projections, acoustic shadows, and ascites.

- Estimate is calculated on
http://www.iotagroup.org/adnexmodel/site%20iota.html

CONCLUSION

- Positive findings for malignancy include **fixed or irregular consistency on pelvic examination, solid or papillary projections on TVS, a serum CA-125 >35 µ/ml, and a PI <1.0 or a RI <0.4 on color Doppler.**
- Study shows that if all four indicators are positive in a postmenopausal woman, the risk for malignancy is 83%. In contrast, if all indicators were negative, 100% of postmenopausal women have benign ovarian tumors.
- Out of four, **tumor morphology index and serum CA-125 are the most significant predictors of malignancy** in the ovarian tumors of postmenopausal women.

INVESTIGATIONS/PREOPERATIVE EVALUATION/WORK-UP

- Workup of undiagnosed pelvic mass is done with an aim to...
  - Confirm malignancy.
  - Determine anatomic location, size, morphology of the tumor, and possible sites of metastases.
  - Detect the primary site.
  - Know general medical condition and ability of patient to undergo a major surgical procedure.

INVESTIGATIONS

- **Routine hematologic** and biochemical testing.

- **Serum markers** according to the age and clinical findings of each patient (e.g., AFP should be considered to assess for germ cell tumors in <35 years with a pelvic mass). (N15)

TUMOR HISTOLOGY	SERUM MARKER
Epithelial ovarian cancer	CA-125
Mucinous cystadenocarcinoma	CEA
Endodermal sinus tumor	AFP
Embryonal cell carcinoma	hCG, AFP
Choriocarcinoma	hCG
Dysgerminoma	LDH-1, LDH-2, PLAP
Granulosa cell tumor	Inhibin

It is important to obtain a baseline serum marker value before surgery so that it can be used to monitor response to therapy.

- **CXR** to know cardiac size and presence of pulmonary metastases or a pleural effusion. **ECG** in older than 40 or in a patient with specific signs or symptoms of cardiac disease.

- **TVS** to assess tumor size and morphology. It is also valuable in identifying intrauterine tumor or occult ascites. A patient with an ovarian tumor and vaginal bleeding should undergo further evaluation to rule out coexisting endometrial cancer or a primary uterine cancer with spread to the ovaries.
- **TAS** in large ovarian tumors with TVS to determine the full extent of the tumor.

- **Abdominal/pelvic CT/MRI** (as clinically indicated) is of limited value for a patient with a definite pelvic mass. A CT or MRI should be performed for

patients with ascites and no pelvic mass to look for liver or pancreatic tumors. (N12, N15) **CECT** may identify ureteral obstruction, retroperitoneal lymphadenopathy, omental disease, liver involvement and peritoneal metastases. It helps in staging of ovarian carcinoma. (T15) CT is useful to assess for metastases. MRI may be useful for determining malignant potential if ultrasound is not reliable. (N15)
- PET/CT scan may be useful for indeterminate lesions. (N15)

- **FNA should be avoided** for diagnosis in presumed early-stage disease to prevent rupturing the cyst and spilling malignant cells into the peritoneal cavity; but may be necessary in patients with bulky disease who are not surgical candidates. (N15)

- **Paracentesis** is contraindicated in a confirmed ovarian tumor on sonography, but it may be useful in a patient who presents with ascites and no evidence of an ovarian abnormality. The characteristics of malignant cells present in ascitic fluid may help to identify the primary site of intraabdominal malignancy.

- **A biopsy** of easily accessible lymph node should be performed.

- **LFT** in a patient with ascites but no ovarian tumor to exclude cirrhosis or liver disease. Rarely, the presence of right heart failure and hepatic congestion will cause ascites.
- **Liver-spleen scans, bone scans and brain scans** are unnecessary unless symptoms or signs suggest metastases to these sites. (N15)

- Value of **Pap test** for the detection of ovarian cancer is not proved.

- Common nongynecologic cancers that spread to the ovary include gastric malignancy, colonic carcinoma, and breast carcinoma. If clinically indicated; evaluate with...
  - **Barium enema or colonoscopy** to rule out colon cancer in presence of occult blood in stool or clinical features of intestinal obstruction.
  - **Upper GI radiographic series or gastroscopy** if there are upper GI symptoms (nausea, vomiting, or hematemesis).
  - **B/L mammography** if there is any breast mass, because occasionally breast cancer metastatic to the ovaries can simulate primary ovarian cancer.
  - **Endometrial biopsy and endocervical curettage** in presence of irregular menses or postmenopausal bleeding to exclude uterine or endocervical cancer metastatic to the ovary.

- A **karyotype** should be obtained preoperatively for all premenarcheal girls because of the propensity of germ cell **tumors to arise in dysgenetic gonads.** **(N12)**

DIFFERENTIAL DIAGNOSIS

- Gynecologic causes...
  - **Pregnancy (young women)**
  - **PID**
  - Ovarian
    - Benign neoplasms and functional cysts
    - Endometriosis
  - Uterine
    - Uterine cancer
    - Pedunculated uterine leiomyomas

- Nongynecologic causes...
  - Inflammatory (e.g., diverticular disease)
  - Neoplastic (colon cancers, pancreatic cancers, lymphoma)
  - A pelvic kidney
  - Acute appendicitis (rare)

2014 FIGO STAGING SYSTEM AND CORRESPONDING TNM

Stage I T1-N0-M0	Tumor confined to ovaries or fallopian tube(s)
IA T1a-N0-M0	Tumor limited to one ovary (capsule intact) or fallopian tube; no tumor on ovarian or fallopian tube surface; no malignant cells in the ascites or peritoneal washings
IB T1b-N0-M0	Tumor limited to both ovaries (capsules intact) or fallopian tubes; no tumor on ovarian or fallopian tube surface; no malignant cells in the ascites or peritoneal washings
IC T1c-N0-M0	tumor limited to one or both ovaries or fallopian tubes, with any of the following: IC1 (T1c1-N0-M0): surgical spill IC2 (T1c2-N0-M0): capsule ruptured before surgery or tumor on ovarian or fallopian tube surface IC3 (T1c3-N0-M0): malignant cells in the ascites or peritoneal washings
Stage II T2-N0-M0	**Tumor involves one or both ovaries or fallopian tubes with pelvic extension (below pelvic brim) or primary peritoneal cancer**
IIA T2a-N0-M0	extension and/or implants on uterus and/or fallopian tubes and/or ovaries
IIB T2b-N0-M0	extension to other pelvic intraperitoneal tissues
Stage III T1/T2-N1-M0	**Tumor involves one or both ovaries or fallopian tubes, or primary peritoneal cancer, with cytologically or histologically confirmed spread to the peritoneum outside the pelvis and/or metastasis to the retroperitoneal lymph nodes**

IIIA	IIIA1: Positive retroperitoneal lymph nodes only (cytologically or histologically proven)
	    • IIIA1(i) Metastasis up to 10 mm in greatest dimension
	    • IIIA1(ii) Metastasis more than 10 mm in greatest dimension
	IIIA2 (T3a2-N0/N1-M0): microscopic extrapelvic (above the pelvic brim) peritoneal involvement with or without positive retroperitoneal lymph nodes

IIIB T3b-N0/N1-M0	Macroscopic peritoneal metastasis beyond the pelvis up to 2 cm in greatest dimension, with or without metastasis to the retroperitoneal lymph nodes
IIIC T3c-N0/N1-M0	Macroscopic peritoneal metastasis beyond the pelvis more than 2 cm in greatest dimension, with or without metastasis to the retroperitoneal lymph nodes (includes extension of tumor to capsule of liver and spleen without parenchymal involvement of either organ)
Stage IV	**Distant metastasis excluding peritoneal metastases**
IVA	**pleural effusion with positive cytology**
IVB Any T, any N, M1	**parenchymal metastases and metastases to extra-abdominal organs (including inguinal lymph nodes and lymph nodes outside of the abdominal cavity)**

- It is not possible to have stage I peritoneal cancer.

PRIMARY TREATMENT

1. NEOADJUVANT CHEMOTHERAPY & INTERVAL CYTOREDUCTIVE SURGERY

- It is recommended alternative for all patients with advanced epithelial ovarian cancer or for certain subsets, such as those predicted to be suboptimally resected.

- The potential advantage is to operate on a patient with an improved nutritional status, a smaller tumor burden, and superior perioperative risk.

- How to predict the unresectability remains unresolved till now. The principal focus has been on preoperative serum CA-125 or CT appearance of disease. Unfortunately, to date, neither has been accurate enough to be incorporated into standard care. Diagnostic laparoscopy has also been investigated as a tool for assessing respectability; this approach may ultimately prove to be the most practical and accurate method, but further study is indicated.

- Studies of neoadjuvant chemotherapy concluded that...
  - 70-80 % of patients treated with neoadjuvant chemotherapy have partial or complete responses before interval surgery;
  - A high proportion of patients so treated, possibly higher than with primary cytoreductive surgery, are optimally debulked with minimal residual disease; and
  - Surgical morbidity may be reduced compared with primary cytoreductive surgery.

- Before initiation of chemotherapy, the pathologic diagnosis should be confirmed (by FNA, biopsy, or paracentesis). If there are concerns about the histology, a core biopsy can be obtained; minimally invasive techniques may be used to obtain the biopsy.

2. SURGICAL STAGING FOR EARLY STAGE OVARIAN CANCER

- Comprehensive surgical staging of early disease (Laparoscopy)...
  - Entry into abdominal cavity and inspection of pelvic and peritoneal cavity
  - Cytology obtained
  - Affected ovary isolated by identification of infundibulopelvic ligament
  - Ureter identified and isolated
  - Infundibulopelvic ligament cauterized and transected

- Utero-ovarian ligament cauterized and transected
- Ovary placed in endoscopic bag intact and removed through largest trocar site assuring no spilling of ovarian tissue
- Frozen section obtained and if consistent with cancer, then formal staging performed
- Omental biopsy performed by coagulation and transection of dessicated tissue
- Pelvic and paraaortic lymph node dissection is performed bilaterally.
- Multiple peritoneal biopsies performed including both paracolic gutters, pelvic peritoneal surfaces bilaterally, and diaphragm peritoneum

- Staging laparotomy...
- Vertical midline incision
- Evacuation of ascites or multiple cytologic washings
- Complete pelvic & abdominal inspection and palpation
- Resection of ovaries, fallopian tubes, and uterus[a]
- Omentectomy & appendectomy
- Random peritoneal biopsies
- Retroperitoneal lymph node sampling

[a]Exceptions may be made in selected patients who wish to preserve fertility.

- If preoperative evaluation suggests an area of extraabdominal or intrahepatic metastasis, FNAC or needle biopsy of this lesion should be performed.

- Because ovarian cancer frequently spreads to upper abdominal structures, a **vertical midline or paramedian abdominal incision** is recommended to allow adequate access to the upper abdomen. This incision should be extended high enough to remove the primary ovarian tumor with its capsule intact (as rupture of a cystic ovarian malignancy is associated with a poorer prognosis) and to evaluate the stomach, omentum, liver, and undersurface of the diaphragm. (T15)

- When a malignancy is unexpectedly discovered in a **lower transverse incision,** the rectus muscles can be either divided or detached from the symphysis pubis to allow better access to the upper abdomen. If this is not sufficient, the incision can be extended on one side to create a **J incision.** (N12)

- Steps...
- The volume of **ascitic fluid, especially in the pelvic cul-de-sac** should be recorded and **a minimum of 25 mL** should be submitted for cytologic evaluation. (T15)

- In the absence of ascites, separate saline washings should be obtained from the (a) pelvic cul-de-sac, (b) each paracolic gutter, & (c) undersurface of each hemidiaphragm. ~100 mL of saline should be instilled in each of these areas, recovered, and sent for cytologic evaluation.
- The ovarian tumor should be inspected for presence of papillary excrescences on the surface or rupture of the capsule. The contralateral ovary and uterus should be examined for metastasis. The pathways of ovarian tumor should be removed and sent for **frozen-section.** (T15) BSO and hysterectomy should be performed with effort to keep an encapsulated mass intact during removal. For selected patients desiring to preserve fertility, USO may be considered. (N15)
- Careful inspection and palpation of the peritoneal surfaces **and intra-abdominal viscera is performed, proceeding in a clockwise fashion from the cecum** cephalad along the paracolic gutter and the ascending colon to the right kidney, the liver and gallbladder, the right hemidiaphragm, the entrance to the lesser sac at the para-aortic area, across the transverse colon to the left hemidiaphragm, spleen, down the left gutter and the descending colon to the rectosigmoid colon and bladder peritoneum. The small intestine and its mesentery from the Treitz ligament to the cecum should be inspected. (N12)
- **Any suspicious areas or adhesions on the peritoneal surfaces should be biopsied.** If there is no evidence of disease, multiple intraperitoneal biopsies from the peritoneum of the pelvic cul-de-sac, both paracolic gutters, both lateral pelvic walls, the peritoneum over the bladder, the intestinal mesenteries and undersurface of the right hemidiaphragm (scrapping with a tougue depressor for Papanicolaou stain) should be taken. (N15)
- The omentum should be resected from the transverse colon, a procedure called an **infracolic omentectomy.** It is initiated on the underside of the greater omentum, where the peritoneum is incised just a few millimeters away from the transverse colon. The branches of the gastroepiploic vessels are clamped, ligated, and divided, along with all the small branching vessels that feed the infracolic omentum. If the gastrocolic ligament is palpably normal, it does not need to be resected. (N12, N15)
- An infracolic omentectomy should be performed in patients with epithelial ovarian cancer and an omental wedge biopsy taken in patients with germ-cell or stromal tumors. (T15) Infracolic omentectomy is initiated on the underside of the greater omentum, where the peritoneum is just a few millimeters away from the transverse colon.

- **Appendectomy** should be performed in mucinous epithelial ovarian cancers. Primary appendiceal cancers, although rare, commonly spread to the ovaries and usually require right hemicolectomy as part of initial surgical staging. (N12)
- **The retroperitoneal spaces should be explored to evaluate the pelvic and para-aortic lymph nodes** by incision of the peritoneum over the psoas muscles.
    - **Para-aortic lymph node dissection** should be performed by stripping the nodal tissue from the vena cava and the aorta bilaterally to at least the level of the inferior mesenteric artery and preferably to the level of the renal vessels.
    - The preferred method of dissecting **pelvic lymph nodes** is bilateral removal of lymph nodes overlying and anterolateral to the common iliac vessel, overlying and medial to the external iliac vessel, overlying and medial to the hypogastric vessels, and from the obturator fossa at a minimum anterior to the obturator nerve. (N15)
- Operative findings present at staging laparotomy must be carefully documented. Prognosis is related to the site and volume of metastatic tumor, as well as the **amount of residual disease remaining after surgical debulking.** (T15)

3. PRIMARY CYTOREDUCTIVE SURGERY FOR ADVANCED STAGE

- The operation to **remove the primary tumor & as much of the associated metastatic disease as possible is referred to as "debulking" or cytoreductive surgery.** (N12)

- Cytoreductive surgery is the initial treatment for clinical stage II, III, or IV disease. (N15)

- **Cytoreductive surgeries are feasible for 70-90% of patients** & survival is improved when performed by gynecologic oncologists. Each **10% increase in cytoreduction equals a 5.5% increase in median survival.**

- In select patients, minimally invasive procedures may be used to...
    - Assess whether cytoreductive surgery is feasible to achieve maximum cytoreduction and
    - Achieve cytoreduction. (N15)
If clinical judgment indicates that maximum cytoreduction cannot be achieved, neoadjuvant chemotherapy should be considered. (N15)

- **Suboptimal debulking:** residual disease ≥1 cm

- **Optimal debulking**: residual disease <1 cm in maximum diameter or thickness

- The cytoreductive surgery (removal of bulky tumor masses, omental cake and intestinal metastases)...

- **Reduces the volume of ascites present.** Often, ascites will completely disappear after removal of the primary tumor and a large omental cake,
- **Alleviates the nausea and early satiety** (removal of the omental cake),
- **Restores adequate intestinal function** and lead to an improvement in the **overall nutritional status** of the patient, thereby facilitating the patient's ability to tolerate subsequent chemotherapy (removal of the omental cake),
- **Removes areas that are poorly vascularized,** and such areas will be exposed to **suboptimal concentrations of chemotherapeutic agents,**
- **Removes areas that are poorly oxygenated,** so that **radiation therapy,** which requires adequate oxygenation to achieve maximal cell kill, **will be less effective,**
- Results in **smaller residual masses with a relatively higher growth fraction** [Larger tumor masses tend to be composed of a higher proportion of cells that are either non-dividing or in the "resting" phase (i.e., G_0 cells, which are essentially resistant to the therapy). A low growth fraction is characteristic of bulky tumor masses].

- The ability of cytoreductive surgery to influence survival is limited by **the extent of metastases before cytoreduction,** presumably because of the **presence of phenotypically resistant clones of cells in large metastatic masses.**

- **Extensive carcinomatosis, the presence of ascites, and poor tumor grade, even with lesions that measure <5 mm,** may also shorten the survival.

- The **diameter of the largest residual tumor nodule before the initiation of chemotherapy is significantly related to PFS** in advanced ovarian cancer. Quality of life is likely to be significantly enhanced by removal of bulky tumor masses from the pelvis and upper abdomen.

- Tumor cells have **an intrinsic spontaneous mutation rate;** larger tumors that go untreated for an extended period contains cell populations resistant to anticancer agents. Therefore, even after optimal debulking, the small residual tumor masses may still contain drug-resistant cells that preclude ultimate cure.

GOALS OF CYTOREDUCTIVE SURGERY

- **Removal of all of the primary cancer and all metastatic disease.** If not feasible, **reduce the tumor burden by resection of all individual tumors to an optimal status.**

EXPLORATION

- **Supine position** may be sufficient. For extensive pelvic disease in which a rectosigmoid resection may be necessary, **the low lithotomy/semi lithotomy/ski position** should be used.

- A vertical **midline incision** (from pubic symphysis to xiphoid) is employed to gain adequate access.

- On entering the abdomen, follow the initial steps outlined under surgical staging.

- **Evacuate ascitic fluid, if present.** Fluid is submitted for molecular analyses. In massive ascites, give attention to hemodynamic monitoring. (N12) For obvious disease beyond the ovaries, cytologic assessment of ascites and/or lavage specimens will not alter stage or management. (N15)

- Inspect and palpate the **peritoneal cavity and retroperitoneum** thoroughly to assess the extent of the primary tumor and the metastatic disease.

- Assess the feasibility of cytoreductive surgery.

- Findings that may initially dissuade the surgeon from proceeding with aggressive tumor resection & that may decide resectability include...
  - Extensive parenchymal hepatic involvement,
  - Diaphragmatic involvement with extension to the pleural cavity,
  - Extensive disease in porta-hepatis,
  - Extensive infiltration of the small intestinal mesentery, or
  - Bulky nodal disease above the renal vessels.

- Even if minimal residual disease cannot be achieved, debulking of omental (omental cake) and pelvic masses (primary tumor) may relieve production of ascites, reduce pressure on adjacent organs, and allow the patient increased comfort, at least temporarily. Moreover, intestinal resection still may be indicated for relief of impending or true obstruction.

- If optimal status is not considered achievable, extensive bowel and urologic resections are not indicated, except to overcome a bowel obstruction.

OMENTECTOMY

- Advanced epithelial ovarian cancer often completely replaces the omentum, forming an "omental cake" & omentectomy is performed before focusing on the pelvis.

- If the omental tumor is adherent to the parietal peritoneum of the anterior abdominal wall, the pelvic structures, or loops of small intestine, it should be dissected from these structures.

- The omentum is then lifted and pulled gently in the cranial direction, exposing **the attachment of the infracolic omentum to the transverse colon.** The peritoneum is incised to open the appropriate plane, which is developed by **sharp dissection along the serosa of the transverse colon.** Small vessels are ligated with hemoclips.

- If the supracolic omentum is heavily involved with tumor and densely adherent to the transverse colon, it also may be necessary to establish a plane between the greater curvature of the stomach and the omentum by ligating the right and left gastroepiploic arteries and the short gastric branches. Entrance into the lesser sac allows traction on the greater curvature of the stomach and facilitates exposure and transection of the gastric branches of the gastroepiploic arch.

- The **disease in the gastrocolic ligament** can extend to **the hilus of the spleen and splenic flexure of the colon on the left and to the capsule of the liver and the hepatic flexure of the colon on the right.** Usually, the disease does not invade the parenchyma of the liver or spleen and a plane can be found between the tumor and these organs. However, it will occasionally be necessary to perform splenectomy to remove all the omental disease.

PELVIC TUMOR RESECTION

- Any adhesions of small intestine or cecum to the pelvic structures should be lysed.

- Self-retaining retractor (Thompson retractor) is inserted & bowel is packed for adequate exposure.

- Retroperitoneal approach is preferred; if normal pelvic spaces and planes are obliterated by tumor. The **retroperitoneum is entered laterally, along the surface of the psoas muscles,** which avoids the iliac vessels and the ureters. The procedure is initiated by **division of the round ligaments bilaterally** if the uterus is present. The **peritoneal incision is extended cephalad, lateral to the ovarian vessels within the infundibulopelvic ligament, and caudally toward**

the bladder. With careful dissection of loose areolar tissue planes using suction tip, the retroperitoneal space is explored, and the ureter and pelvic vessels are identified. Next, the ovarian vessels are ligated. The identical procedure is performed on the opposite side of the pelvis, and the tumor mass (es) is (are) mobilized medially. The pararectal and paravesicular spaces are identified and developed.

- Dissect & free the entire length of the pelvic portion of the ureter to the uterovesical junction; if the ureters are densely adherent to the pelvic tumor.

- Dissect the plane between the sigmoid colon and the uterus and ovaries. If such dissection is not feasible or that the wall of the colon is heavily infiltrated with tumor (involvement of the lumina of the colon is rare), resection of the rectosigmoid colon may be indicated. Resection of the pelvic portion of the colon allows the surgeon access to the avascular retrorectal space.

- The uterus is dissected from the bladder as well. Involvement of the bladder mucosa is rare **(hematuria if involved, do preoperative cystoscopy)**, but the vesicouterine peritoneum may be heavily infiltrated. The peritoneum overlying the bladder is dissected to connect the peritoneal incisions anteriorly. The vesicouterine plane is identified, and with careful sharp dissection **the bladder is mobilized from the anterior surface of the cervix.** Occasionally partial cystectomy is required to achieve optimal cytoreduction. (N12)

- Total hysterectomy is then performed, the vagina is entered, and the mass is removed en bloc. It may be necessary to ligate the uterine vessels at their origin rather than near the uterus if tumor is extensive in this area. Also, supracervical hysterectomy may be advisable if there is extensive unresectable tumor in the cul-de-sac. (N12, N15)

INTESTINAL RESECTION

- The disease may involve **focal areas of the small or large intestine and resection should be performed** if it would permit the removal of all or most of the abdominal metastases and the patient will be left with optimal disease at the end of the cytoreduction. **The most frequent sites of intestinal metastasis are rectosigmoid colon (MC site), the terminal ileum, the cecum, and the transverse colon.** Resection of one or more of these segments of bowel may be necessary.

- If the disease **surrounds the rectosigmoid colon and its mesentery**, it may be necessary to remove that portion of the colon to clear the pelvic disease (in 10% of patients during primary debulking).

- The decision depends on...
  - The presence or absence of rectosigmoid obstruction,
  - The amount of tumor infiltration of the lower colon and its contiguity with the ovarian tumor(s), and
  - The probability that such a procedure will render the patient optimally debulked.

- In the presence of unresectable bulky residual tumor in the upper abdomen or retroperitoneum; palliative resection in the absence of obstruction is not recommended.

- After the pararectal space is identified in such patients, the proximal site of colonic involvement is identified, the colon and its mesentery are divided, and the rectosigmoid is removed along with the uterus en bloc.

- In most cases the colon can be reanastomosed using either a suture technique or the end-to-end anastomosis (EEA) stapler. For patients who undergo a reanastomosis, a protective hepatic flexure transverse loop colostomy or loop ileostomy protects the anastomosis for those who have received pelvic radiotherapy, those with unprepared colon, or those whose anastomosis is judged to be suboptimal. Occasionally, a colostomy with a Hartmann's pouch is necessary.

- If the **small intestine** is extensively involved with tumor, it is usually in the terminal ileum.
- Indications for small intestinal resection include (in 5-10% of patients during primary debulking)...
  - Obstruction or impending obstruction by tumor infiltrating the serosa and muscularis of a segment or
  - A nonobstructing extensive lesion of the small intestine for which resection would result in minimal residual disease.

- If the lesion involves the very terminal portion of the ileum, an ileocolectomy with resection of the cecum and portion of ascending colon adjacent to the small intestine may be necessary. Care should be taken to avoid the presence of tumor at the points of reanastomosis. The reanastomosis may be performed using either the suture or the stapling technique.

- Intestinal resection in these patients doesn't appear to increase overall morbidity.

RESECTION OF URINARY TRACT

- Indications for ureteral resection or partial cystectomy are uncommon. If ureteral obstruction is noted preoperatively, it is almost always a result of ureteral compression rather than tumor infiltration.

- If distal ureter is resected, reimplant it into bladder.

- If the ureter is injured; depending on the site of injury, a primary reanastomosis, transureteroureterostomy, or ureteroneocystostomy may be indicated.

- Tumor involvement of the peritoneum overlying bladder is not an uncommon finding. Partial cystectomy may be necessary to achieve optimal cytoreduction. A simple closure with 2 layers of chromic catgut, inner layer as a continuous running and outer layer as interrupted sutures is preferred.

SPLENECTOMY (5-11% of advanced ovarian cancer)

- Most commonly, the hilum of the spleen is involved with ovarian cancer in association with extensive omental involvement.
- Splenectomy may be indicated because of...
  - Traction injury with avulsion of the splenic capsule during omentectomy or
  - Mobilization of the splenic flexure of the colon in association with descending colostomy or
  - Reanastomosis after rectosigmoid colon resection.

- Rarely, isolated splenic capsular involvement or even splenic parenchymal involvement may be found.
  - Under controlled conditions (no uncontrolled hemorrhage), the surgeon may prefer to incise the gastrosplenic ligament, gain access to the lesser sac, and identify and ligate the splenic vessels as they run along the superior border of the pancreas. The spleen then can be mobilized by transecting its attachments to the colon, the left kidney, and the diaphragm.
  - If hemorrhage is occurring or access to the lesser sac is limited by the distribution of tumor, the surgeon may prefer to first mobilize the spleen by dividing its peritoneal attachments while compressing the splenic vessels, and then ligate the splenic vessels using a posterior approach. The spleen is rotated anteriorly and medially in this technique.

- Complications...
  - Hemorrhage,
  - Infection,
  - Thromboembolic phenomena,
  - Left-sided atelectasis or pneumonia,
  - Injury to the tail of the pancreas (with resultant pancreatic pseudocyst), or
  - Injury to the stomach (with resultant gastric fistula).

- Perioperative antibiotic coverage and vaccination with polyvalent pneumococcal, quadrivalent meningococcal, and hemophilus influenzae vaccines is must.

RESECTION OF DIAPHRAGMATIC TUMOR

- The abdominal incision is extended to just below the xiphoid process, and the liver is mobilized by transecting the entire falciform ligament and the coronary and triangular ligaments.

- The diaphragmatic tumor may be resected by stripping the peritoneum from the diaphragmatic muscle using sharp dissection with either Metzenbaum scissors or electrocautery.

- Defects in the diaphragm may be closed with interrupted sutures. If a large defect cannot be closed primarily or can be closed only under tension, then the defect may be closed using synthetic mesh. If the pleural cavity is entered, then a thoracostomy tube should be placed.

- Complications...
  • Pneumothorax,
  • Hemorrhage from the phrenic arteries,
  • Infection,
  • Injury to the pericardial sac, and
  • Injury to such structures as the lung, the vena cava, or the phrenic nerves.

RESECTION OF OTHER METASTASES & LYMPH NODE

- Other large isolated masses of tumor **located on the parietal peritoneum** should be removed, particularly if their **removal will permit optimal cytoreduction.** The use of the **Cavitron Ultrasonic Surgical Aspirator (CUSA), Nd-YAG laser** and **the argon beam coagulator** may help facilitate resection of small tumor nodules, especially those on flat surfaces. (N12)

- Suspicious and/or enlarged nodes should be resected, if possible. Bilateral pelvic and para-aortic lymph node dissection is recommended for those patients with tumor nodules, outside the pelvis, of 2 cm or less (presumed stage IIIB). (N15)

OPERATIVE NOTES

- Extent of initial disease before debulking pelvis, mid-abdomen, or upper abdomen (cutoffs: pelvic brim to lower ribs).
- Amount of residual disease in the same after debulking.
- Complete or incomplete resection; if incomplete, indicate the size of the major lesion and total number of lesions. Indicate if miliary or small lesions.

4. POST OPERATIVE CHEMOTHERAPY/ADJUVANT CHEMOTHERAPY

- Postoperative chemotherapy (primary chemotherapy) is beneficial in the patients at risk for relapse after primary surgery.

MALIGNANT GERM CELL TUMORS: Postop chemoRx of BEP regime is required in all malignant germ cell tumors except stage I pure dysgerminoma & stage I grade 1 immature teratoma.

SEX CORD STROMAL TUMORS: Postop chemoRx of BEP regime or paclitaxel + carboplatin combination is required in...
- o   Stage II-IV, and
- o   Stage I high risk (e.g., rupture, IC, poorly differentiated, tumor size >10-15 cm) or intermediate risk (heterologus elements).

INVASIVE EPITHELIAL TUMORS: Postop chemoRx is indicated in...
- o   Early-stage EOC with high risk features
- o   Advanced-stage EOC.

EARLY-STAGE EPITHELIAL OVARIAN CANCER RISK GROUPS	
Low Risk	**High Risk**
- Stage IA or IB, grade 1 and 2	- Stage IA or IB, grade 3 - Stage IC - All stage II - Ascites/positive peritoneal washing - Dense adherence - Clear-cell histology - Tumor on external surface - Capsule rupture
- The standard treatment is surgery alone, and the 5-year survival is at least 95%.	- This group has a relapse risk of 40-50% and is the focus of adjuvant therapy trials.

BORDERLINE TUMOR: Borderline tumors with invasive peritoneal implants have life time risk for relapse around 50%. Consequently, postoperative platinum-based chemotherapy is recommended (benefit not proved).

MAINTENANCE THERAPY

- Since 70% or more patients with advanced epithelial ovarian cancer ultimately develop disease recurrence, the strategy of maintenance or consolidation therapy after completion of primary chemotherapy has been studied in an effort to decrease the relapse rate. See in management of EOC.

SECONDARY SURGERY

SECOND LOOK OPERATIONS

- It was done in patients after primary treatment **to determine the response to therapy & disease status. It is obsolete.**

(A) SECOND-LOOK LAPAROTOMY

- The technique is identical to that for the staging laparotomy.

- Performed through a **vertical abdominal incision.** The incision should be initiated below the level of the umbilicus, so that if pelvic disease is detected in the absence of any palpable upper abdominal disease, a smaller incision might suffice. The incision can be extended cranially as needed.

- After **multiple cytologic specimens** have been obtained, samples of the peritoneal surfaces should be collected for **biopsy, particularly in any areas of previously documented tumor.** These are the most important areas to sample for biopsy because they are most likely to give a positive result. Any **adhesions or surface irregularities should be sampled.** In addition, biopsy specimens should be taken from the pelvic side walls, the pelvic cul-de-sac, the bladder, the paracolic gutters, the residual omentum, and the diaphragm.

- A **pelvic and para-aortic lymph node dissection** should be performed for those patients whose nodal tissues have not been previously removed.

- ~**30% of patients with no evidence of macroscopic disease** will have microscopic metastases. Also, for many patients with microscopic disease, it will be detected in only the occasional biopsy or cytologic specimen. Therefore, a **large number of specimens (at least 20-30) should be obtained** to minimize possibility of false-negative results of the operation. In selected patients in whom gross residual tumor is discovered at second-look surgery, resection of isolated masses may be performed. The removal of all macroscopic areas of disease might facilitate response to salvage therapies.

INDICATION:

- It has **not been shown to influence survival.** So perform **selectively,** e.g., in patients receiving therapy in a setting where second-line therapies are undergoing clinical trials.

CLINICAL IMPORTANCE:

- The **findings** at second-look **correlate with subsequent outcome and survival.** Patients who have no histologic evidence of disease have a significantly longer survival than those in whom microscopic or macroscopic disease is documented at laparotomy. The **attainment of negative findings with second-look surgery is not tantamount to a cure.** Indeed, **the probability that a patient will have a recurrence after a negative second-look laparotomy ranges from 30-50% at 5 years.** Clearly, it is not possible to sample every potential site of disease. In addition, disease can become clinically apparent in sites that are occult, such as the liver parenchyma. **Most recurrences after a negative second-look laparotomy occur in patients with poorly differentiated cancers.**

- Findings at second-look surgery are classified as...
- Negative (grossly and pathologically negative) (30-50%),
- Microscopically positive (grossly negative, pathologically positive) (20%), and
- Macroscopically positive (grossly and pathologically positive) (30-50%).

Factors affecting findings of second look laparotomy are (i) initial stage, (ii) tumor grade, (iii) the size of the residual tumor and the size of the largest metastatic tumor before treatment, and (iv) the type of chemotherapy. No single variable or combination of variables is sufficiently predictive of the findings of a second-look laparotomy.

(B) SECOND-LOOK LAPAROSCOPY

- In epithelial ovarian cancer may be used...
- To stage disease in patients who have undergone a prior laparotomy for a tumor that was incompletely staged.
- For patients on experimental treatment protocols, especially second-line treatments that require some evaluation of response.

- The **advantage of laparoscopy is that it is a less invasive operation; the disadvantage is that visibility may be limited by the frequent presence of intraperitoneal adhesions.**

SECONDARY CYTOREDUCTIVE SURGERY

- An **attempt at cytoreductive surgery who have developed recurrent disease at some stage following completion of first-line chemotherapy.**

- In patients...

(a) Who are partial responders or nonresponders to primary chemotherapy,

(b) Who have developed recurrent disease after receiving primary therapy and experience a prolonged disease-free interval off therapy (>6 months) (most common),

(c) Who undergo a suboptimal debulking initially followed by three cycles of chemotherapy (so-called interval debulking), and,

(d) Who have persistent macroscopic tumor at second-look laparotomy.

- The principal setting for secondary cytoreductive surgery is for platinum-sensitive recurrent disease. Patients with **progressive disease on chemotherapy are not suitable candidates** for secondary cytoreduction.

- Tumor resection under these circumstances **should be restricted to those who have a disease-free interval of at least 12, but preferably 24, months or those in whom all macroscopic disease can be resected, regardless of the disease free interval.** Complete resection is possible when there are only one or two isolated recurrences in patient without diffuse carcinomatosis.

TERTIARY CYTOREDUCTIVE SURGERY

- Treatment free interval before tertiary cytoreduction, the extent of residual disease after the procedure, and the time to first recurrence are significant prognostic factors. Multivariate analysis identified platinum resistance, tumor residuals at secondary surgery, and peritoneal carcinomatosis to be of predictive significance for complete tumor resection, while tumor residuals at secondary and tertiary surgery, decreasing interval to second relapse, ascites, upper abdominal tumor involvement, and nonplatinum third-line chemotherapy significantly affect overall survival.

EPITHELIAL OVARIAN CARCINOMA

INTRODUCTION/EPIDEMIOLOGY

- EOC is the leading cause of death from gynecologic cancer in the US and is the country's fifth MC cause of cancer mortality in women.

- Epithelial cancers are the **MC ovarian malignancies**, and because they are usually asymptomatic until they have metastasized, patients have advanced disease at diagnosis in >2/3 of the cases.

ORIGIN

- ~**90%** of ovarian cancers are derived from the **coelomic epithelium or mesothelium**. The cells are a product of the **primitive mesoderm**, which can undergo metaplasia. (N12)

TYPES

BENIGN

- Not explained here.

BORDERLINE TUMORS (TUMOR OF LOW MALIGNANT POTENTIAL)

- Occur predominantly **in premenopausal** women; between **30-50 years. Average age is ~46 years.**
- Remain **confined to the ovary** for long periods.
- A **very good prognosis.** (N12)

INVASIVE CARCINOMAS

- Most frequently in between **50-70 years.**

CLASSIFICATION

HISTOLOGIC TYPE	CELLULAR TYPE	INCIDENCE
1. Serous or Papillary • benign • borderline • malignant	**Endosalpingeal;** glandular epithelial lining of fallopian tube.	75%
2. Mucinous • benign • borderline • malignant	Endocervical; resembles the **endocervical glands,** but more commonly these cells resemble the GI epithelium.	20%
3. Endometroid • benign • borderline • malignant	Endometrial; resembles the proliferative **enodmetrium.**	6-8%
4. Clear-cell mesonephroid • benign • borderline • malignant	**Mullerian; resembles secretory or gestational endometrium.**	<1%
5. Brenner • benign • borderline • malignant	**Transitional;** resembles to the epithelium in Walthard rests & bladder urothelium.	<1%
6. Mixed epithelial • Benign • Borderline • Malignant	Mixed.	
7. Undifferentiated	Anaplastic.	<1%
8. Unclassified	Mesothelioma, etc.	

1. SEROUS TUMORS (75% OF ALL EPITHELIAL TUMORS)

- Serous tumors develop by invagination of the surface epithelium and are so classified because they secrete serous fluid (as do tubal secretory cells).

- Serous epithelial ovarian cancers are separated into...

TYPE I	TYPE II
Serous borderline tumors & low grade serous carcinoma.	Rapidly growing, highly aggressive, lacks well defined precursor lesions; most are advanced stage at, or soon after, their inception and many appear to **arise in the fimbrial end of the fallopian tube.**
Genetically stable.	Genetically unstable.
Mutation in KRAS & BRAF.	Mutation in p53.

- **Psammoma bodies...**
  - Foci of foreign material frequently are associated with these invaginations and may be a response to irritative agents that produce adhesion formation and the entrapment of the surface epithelium.
  - Apoptosis of tumor cells and osteoinductive cytokines produced by macrophages may be responsible.
  - Made up of concentric rings of calcification.

- In the wall of the mesothelial invaginations, **papillary ingrowths** are common, representing the early stages of development of a **papillary serous cystadenoma**. There are many variations in the proliferation of these mesothelial inclusions. Several foci may be lined with flattened inactive epithelium; in adjacent cavities, papillary excrescences are present, often resulting from local irritants.

BORDERLINE OR LOW MALIGNANT POTENTIAL SEROUS TUMORS (10% OF ALL SEROUS TUMORS)

- 50% occur before 40 years.

- **The criteria for the diagnosis of serous borderline tumors:**
  - Epithelial hyperplasia in the form of pseudostratification, tufting, cribriform, and micropapillary architecture.
  - Mild nuclear atypia and mild increased mitotic activity.
  - Detached cell clusters.

- Absence of destructive stromal invasion (i.e., without tissue destruction).

Serous borderline tumors with exuberant micropapillary architecture are more frequently bilateral, exophytic and high stage than the usual serous borderline tumor. (N12)

- Although uncommon, 40% of serous borderline tumors are associated with spread (implants) beyond the ovary, but it does not necessarily warrant a diagnosis of carcinoma. The diagnosis of a serous borderline tumor versus serous carcinoma is based on the histologic features of the primary tumor. The implants are divided histologically into...

- 10% of serous borderline tumors with extraovarian implants may have **invasive implants** and behave more aggressively (high chances of developing into progressive, proliferative disease in the peritoneal cavity, which can lead to intestinal obstruction and death). The 5 year survival is ~50%. The invasive implants resemble well-differentiated serous carcinoma and are characterized by atypical cells forming irregular glands with sharp borders.

- Most implants are **noninvasive**. In noninvasive implants, papillary proliferations of atypical cells involve the peritoneal surface and form smooth invaginations. (N12)

Implants are usually confined to the abdominal cavity & may be seen in the pelvis, omentum, and adjacent tissues, including lymph nodes; metastases outside the abdominal cavity are rare. Death can occur as the result of intestinal obstruction. (N12)

- Serous borderline tumors may harbor **foci of stromal microinvasion.** Most patients are young and FIGO stage I. Stromal microinvasion is increased about ninefold in pregnant women with serous borderline tumors. The presence of stromal microinvasion is **associated with LVSI in the primary ovarian tumor** & likely represents a form of true stromal invasion, but it is not associated with an aggressive clinical course, and patients with this finding should be managed in the **same way as patients without stromal microinvasion.** (N12)

MALIGNANT SEROUS CARCINOMAS

- Stromal invasion is present.

- The grade of tumor should be identified...

- **In well-differentiated (low grade),** papillary and glandular structures predominate.
- **In poorly differentiated (high grade),** solid sheets of cells, nuclear pleomorphism, and high mitotic activity predominate.
- **Moderately differentiated** carcinomas are intermediate between these two. (N12)

- **Laminated, calcified psammoma bodies** are found in 80% of serous carcinomas. (N12)

- **Serous psammocarcinoma** is a rare variant of serous carcinoma characterized by massive psammoma body formation and low-grade cytological features. At least 75% of the epithelial nests are associated with psammoma body formation. Patients with serous psammocarcinoma have a protracted clinical course and a relatively favorable prognosis; their clinical course more closely resembles that of high stage, progressive serous borderline tumor than serous carcinoma. (N12)

2. MUCINOUS TUMORS (20% OF ALL EPITHELIAL TUMORS)

- These cystic ovarian tumors have loculi lined with mucin-secreting epithelium. The lining epithelial cells contain intracytoplasmic mucin and resemble those of **endocervix, gastric pylorus, or intestine.**
- They may reach enormous size, filling the entire abdominal cavity. (N12)

BORDERLINE OR LOW MALIGNANT POTENTIAL MUCINOUS TUMORS

- Difficult to diagnose as it is common to find a uniform pattern from section to section in the serous borderline tumor but not in the mucinous tumors.

- Frequently, **well-differentiated mucinous epithelium may be seen immediately adjacent to a poorly differentiated focus.** Therefore, it is **important to take multiple sections from many areas in the mucinous tumor to identify the most malignant alteration.** (N12)

MALIGNANT MUCINOUS CARCINOMAS

- **Bilateral tumors occur in 8-10% of cases.** The mucinous lesions are intraovarian in 95-98% of cases. **Because most ovarian mucinous carcinomas contain intestinal-type cells, they cannot be distinguished from metastatic carcinoma of the gastrointestinal tract on the basis of histology alone.**

- Primary ovarian neoplasms rarely metastasize to the mucosa of the bowel, although they commonly involve the serosa, whereas gastrointestinal lesions frequently involve the ovary by direct extension of vascular lymphatic spread. (N12)

PSEUDOMYXOMA PERITONEI

- It is used to describe the finding of abundant mucoid or gelatinous material in the pelvis and abdominal cavity surrounded by fibrous tissue. It is most commonly secondary to a **well-differentiated appendiceal mucinous** neoplasm or **other gastrointestinal primary;** rarely, mucinous tumors arising in an ovarian mature teratoma are associated with pseudomyxoma peritonei. (N12)

3. ENDOMETROID TUMORS (6-8% OF ALL EPITHELIAL TUMORS)

- Endometroid neoplasia includes all the benign demonstrations of **endometriosis.** Some cases of adenocarcinoma of the ovary arise in areas of endometriosis, **similar to those seen in the uterine corpus.** The malignant potential of endometriosis is very low, although a transition from benign to malignant epithelium may be demonstrated.

- Endometroid carcinoma is associated with **endometrial carcinoma in 20% & ovarian endometriosis in 10%** of cases. In **less than 5%,** it may arise from the endometrial cyst.

BORDERLINE OR LOW MALIGNANT POTENTIAL ENDOMETROID TUMORS

- It has a wide morphologic spectrum ranging from an endometrial polyp to complex endometrial hyperplasia with glandular crowding.

- When there are back-to-back glands, architecturally complex glands with no intervening stroma, the tumor is classified as a **well-differentiated endometroid carcinoma.**

- Borderline endometroid tumor with fibromatous component is **adenofibroma.**

MALIGNANT ENDOMETROID CARCINOMAS

- Endometroid tumors are characterized by a markedly complex glandular pattern **with all the potential variations of epithelia** found in the uterus.

MULTIFOCAL DISEASE

- **Endometroid carcinoma of the ovary is associated in 15-20% of the cases with carcinoma of the endometrium.** Identification of multifocal disease is important, because patients with disease metastatic from the uterus to the ovaries have a **30-40% 5-year survival,** whereas those with synchronous multifocal disease have a **75% to 80% 5-year survival.**

- **When the histologic appearance of endometrial and ovarian tumors is different,** the two tumors most likely represent two separate primary lesions. **When they appear similar,** the endometrial tumor can be considered a separate primary tumor if it is well differentiated and only superficially invasive.

4. CLEAR CELL CARCINOMAS

- Several basic histologic patterns are present in the clear cell adenocarcinoma (i.e., tubulocystic, papillary, recticular, and solid). The tumors are made up of **clear and hobnail cells** that project their nuclei to the apical cytoplasm.

- The tall clear cells have **abundant clear or vacuolated cytoplasm, hyperchromatic irregular nuclei, and nucleoli** of various sizes. **Focal areas of endometriosis are common and mixed clear cell and endometrioid carcinoma may occur.**

- Histologically **identical to clear cell carcinoma of uterus or vagina of the young patient who has been exposed to DES in utero.**

- Pure grade 1 tumors are extremely rare. **Almost invariably high-grade (grade 3) nuclei are identified. Hence, clear cell carcinoma is not graded.**

5. BRENNER/TRANSITIONAL TUMORS

BORDERLINE OR PROLIFERATING OR LOW MALIGNANT POTENTIAL BRENNER TUMORS

- In such cases, the epithelium does not invade the stroma.

- Subclassification...
- Those tumors that resembles low-grade papillary urothelial carcinoma of the urinary bladder as **proliferating tumors** and
- Those with a high grade papillary urothelial carcinoma as **borderline malignant Brenner tumors.**

- Complete surgical removal usually results in cure.

MALIGNANT BRENNER TUMORS

- These rare tumors are defined as **benign or borderline Brenner tumors coexisting with invasive transitional cells or another carcinoma.** In malignant Brenner tumors there is stromal invasion associated with a benign or borderline Brenner tumor component.

6. MIXED EPITHELIAL

7. UNDIFFERENTIATED

8. MESOTHELIOMAS

- Peritoneal malignant mesotheliomas fall into the following four categories...
      (i) Fibrosarcomatous,
      (ii) Tubulopapillary (papillary-alveolar),
      (iii) Carcinomatous, and
      (iv) Mixed.

- Peritoneal malignant mesotheliomas may be **epithelial, sarcomatous or biphasic.** Decidual peritoneal mesothelioma is an unusual variant that resembles exuberant, ectopic decidual reaction of the peritoneum.

- Asbestos exposure is not correlated with peritoneal mesotheliomas in women.

- These lesions appear as multiple intraperitoneal masses; often coating the entire peritoneum and **can develop after hysterectomy and BSO** for benign disease. Malignant mesotheliomas should be distinguished from benign multicystic peritoneal mesothelioma (multilocular peritoneal inclusion cyst), ovarian tumor implants and primary peritoneal mullerian neoplasms.

9. OTHERS

(I) TRANSITIONAL CELL CARCNOMA

- The designation transitional cell carcinoma refers to a **primary ovarian carcinoma resembling transitional cell carcinoma of the urinary bladder without a recognizable Brenner tumor.**

- Ovarian carcinomas that contain >50% of transitional cell carcinoma are more sensitive to chemotherapy and have a more favorable prognosis than other poorly differentiated ovarian carcinomas of comparable stage.

- **Transitional cell tumors differ from malignant Brenner tumors in that they are more frequently diagnosed in an advanced stage and, therefore, are associated with a poorer survival rate.**

(II) SMALL CELL CARCINOMA

- It occurs mainly in young women, who may have symptoms of **hypercalcemia.** Immunohistochemical stains are helpful to differentiate this tumor from a lymphoma, leukemia, or sarcoma.

(III) PERITONEAL CARCINOMAS

- Primary peritoneal tumors are histologically **indistinguishable from primary ovarian serous tumors.**

- In the case of borderline serous peritoneal tumors and serous peritoneal carcinomas, the ovaries are normal or minimally involved, and the tumors affect **predominantly the USL, pelvic peritoneum, or omentum.**

- The overall **prognosis for borderline serous peritoneal tumors is excellent** and comparable to that of ovarian borderline serous tumors.

- **Carcinoma that appears predominantly as peritoneal carcinomatosis without appreciable ovarian or fallopian tube enlargement is called peritoneal carcinoma or mullerian carcinoma when tumors spread from breast, GI tract and other organs of nonmullerian origin are excluded.** Peritoneal serous carcinomas have the appearance of a moderately to poorly differentiated serous ovarian carcinoma. Primary peritoneal endometrioid carcinoma is less common.

- The primary malignant transformation of the peritoneum has been called primary peritoneal carcinoma or **primary peritoneal papillary serous carcinoma.** Peritoneal carcinoma simulates ovarian & fallopian tube cancer clinically. In patients for whom exploratory surgery is performed, there may be microscopic or small macroscopic cancer on the surface of the ovary and extensive disease in the upper abdomen, particularly in the omentum. This phenomenon can thus produce a condition in which so-called ovarian cancer can arise in a patient whose ovaries were surgically removed many years earlier. Staging & treatment is same as epithelial ovarian carcinoma.

PATHOLOGY

- These tumors are bilateral in 50% of cases. Cystic is more common than solid. These may arise de novo as malignant or more commonly, they result from malignant changes of benign cystic tumors.

CYSTIC

Naked eye appearances- The wall of the cystic tumor becomes shaggy. There may be papillary projection at places. Cut section shows solid areas with hemorrhage at places. The papillae become friable; the base becomes broad and indurated. In mucinous type, it is filled up with gelatinous material.

Microscopic picture-

Type of tumor	Histologic picture
Serous cyst carcinoma	Adenocarcinoma
Mucinous cyst carcinoma	
Endometroid or Adenoacanthoma	
Malignant dermoid	Squamous cell carcinoma

SOLID

Naked eye appearances- It attains a moderate size. The external surface is smooth & often lobulated. Subserous blood vessels may be prominent. Cut section shows grayish granular appearance, at times brain like. There may be irregular cystic spaces due to necrosis.

Microscopic picture- reveals adenocarcinoma or carcinoma without adenomatous pattern.

ETIOLOGY & RISK FACTORS

1) AGE:

- ~**30% of ovarian epithelial tumors in postmenopausal are malignant,** whereas only ~**7% of ovarian epithelial tumors in premenopausal patients are frankly malignant.** (N12)

- **>80% of epithelial ovarian cancers are found in postmenopausal women,** rare before 40 years.

- The chance that a primary epithelial tumor will be of borderline or invasive malignancy in <40 years is ~1 in 10, but after that age it rises to 1 in 3.
- <1% of epithelial ovarian cancers occur before 21 years, 2/3rd of ovarian malignancies in them are germ cell tumors.
- The age specific incidence ↑ses steadily & peaks in the 6th and 7th decades of life (median age 63 years) and subsequently declines. (N15)

2) PARITY:

- Most important nongenetic factor. (T15)
- **Low parity, infertility, older age (>35 years) at pregnancy and first birth** ↑ses risk.
- Parity $\propto$ 1/the risk of ovarian cancer. Risk ↓ses significantly with each term pregnancy. Having at least one child is protective, **with a risk reduction of 0.3-0.4.** (N12)
- Risk decreases with younger age at pregnancy and first birth (≤25 years). (N15)

3) THEORY OF INCESSANT OVULATION:

- **Risk of epithelial ovarian cancer $\propto$ Number of uninterrupted ovulatory cycles.**

Ovulation

Surface epithelium is ruptured

Surface epithelium undergoes rapid proliferation & repair

Invagination of surface epithelium into the underlying stroma forming inclusion cysts

Epithelium lining these inclusion cysts undergoes neoplastic transformation under the influence of oncogenic factors or this process might lead to a higher probability of spontaneous mutations that can unmask germline mutations

- **Early menarche and late menopause** ↑ses risk by ↑sing the number of ovulatory cycles.
- No breast feeding ↑ses risk.

4) RETROGRADE MENSTRUATION HYPOTHESIS:

Menstruation
↓
Retrograde transportation of carcinogens from the uterus & lower genital tract
↓
Fallopian tube
↓
Ovary

- **OCP use** ↓**ses risk (epithelial ovarian cancer)** ~10% per year to ~50% after 5 years of use by…↓se in menstrual blood loss and therefore with ↓sed retrograde menstruation & by decreasing ovulatory cycles.
- **Tubal ligation or hysterectomy** ↓**se risk** by preventing the ascent of oncogenic factors to the ovary.
- **HRT** ↑**ses risk** through the periods of abnormal uterine bleeding.

5) EXPOSURE OF OVARIAN EPITHELIUM TO PERSISTENTLY HIGH LEVELS OF PITUITARY GONADOTROPINS RESULTS IN NEOPLASTIC TRANSFORMATION:

Fertility drugs (ovulation induction) for IVF
↓
Pituitary
↓
↑se FSH
↓
Promote estrogen biosynthesis in the ovarian stroma
↓
Abnormal proliferation of the adjacent epithelium
↓
↑se the growth of EOC & LMP tumors

- This effect can be blocked by LH.
- **Breast-feeding, pregnancy and OCP** ↓**se the risk** by inhibiting pituitary secretion of gonadotropins.

6) FAMILY HISTORY (GENETICS & OVARIAN MALIGNANCY) (15%):

- **Most important risk factor for epithelial ovarian cancer.**

- Hereditary ovarian cancers, particularly those caused by BRCA1 mutations, occur in women 10 years younger than those with nonhereditary tumors. (N12)

- Because the median age of epithelial ovarian cancer is in the mid- to late 50s, a woman with a first- or second-degree relative who had premenopausal ovarian cancer may have a higher probability of carrying an affected gene. (N12)

	OR	LR
Without family history		1.4%
1 first-degree relative	3.1	5%
≥2 first or second degree relatives	4.6	7%

HEREDITARY/FAMILIAL OVARIAN CANCER **(15%)**

AUTOSOMAL DOMINANT (INHERITANCE RISK 50%)		
HBOC (75-90%) (MC)	**HSSOC (5%)**	**HNPCC/LYNCH SYNDROME II**
Multiple cases of early-onset (<50 years of age) breast and ovarian cancers.	Increase in cases of early-onset ovarian cancer. Women are younger and more commonly have tumors with _serous histology_.	Predominance of early-onset proximal colon cancer with endometrial **(LR-50%)** & ovarian carcinoma **(LR-10-12%)**.
Germline mutations in the BRCA1 or BRCA2 gene appear to account for most hereditary ovarian cancers. 1) BRCA1 (80-90%) (1994) (17q) (LR-39%) is tumour suppressor. 2) BRCA2 (10-20%) (1995) (13q) (LR-11%). The **risk of breast cancer** in women with a BRCA1 or BRCA2 mutation may be as high as **56-87%**.		Mutation in mismatch-repair genes, MLH1, PMS1, PMS2, MSH2, and MSH6. LR of ovarian cancer in women with HNPCC is 10-12%. RR of ovarian cancer in women with HNPCC is 3 times the RR of the general population.

- **Founder Effect:** There is a higher carrier rate of BRCA1 and BRCA2 mutations in Ashkenazi Jewish descent and in Icelandic women. 3 specific mutations are carried by the Ashkenazi population, 185delAG and 5382insC on BRCA1, and 6174 delT on BRCA2. The total carrier rate for a patient of Ashkenazi Jewish descent to have **at least one of these three mutations is 1 in 40, or 2.5%,** and thus there is a substantial risk in this population. The increased risk is a result of the **founder effect, in which a higher rate of mutations occurs in an ethnic group from a defined geographic area.**

7) EPIDEMIOLOGIC VARIABLES:

- **Talc use and galactose consumption** increase the risk of ovarian cancer. (N12)

8) BENIGN GYNECOLOGICAL CONDITIONS:

- PID. (N15)

PATTERNS OF SPREAD

- The specific pattern of spread depends on the stage, cell type, and histologic differentiation of the tumor.

1. TRANSCOELOMIC

- **MC and earliest mode of dissemination** of ovarian epithelial cancer that implant along the surfaces of the peritoneal cavity by...
  - Direct exfoliation of cells as in papillary cyst adenocarcinoma.
  - Penetration of tumor capsule.
  - Rupture of the capsule.

- The cells follow the circulatory path of the peritoneal fluid → move with the forces of respiration from the pelvis, up the paracolic gutters, **especially on the right**, along the intestinal mesenteries, to the right hemidiaphragm. Spread to the right lung occurs through the transdiaphragmatic lymphatics in the right hemidiaphragm, often producing a right pleural effusion. Metastases are typically seen on the posterior cul-de-sac, paracolic gutters, right hemidiaphragm, liver capsule, peritoneal surfaces of the intestines and their mesenteries, bladder surface and the omentum.

- The disease seldom invades bowel lumen & bladder mucosa but progressively agglutinates loops of bowel, leading to a functional intestinal obstruction. This condition is known as **carcinomatous ileus**.

2. LYMPHATIC

- Common in advanced-stage disease.

- Follows two pathways...
  - The first involves **lateral spread through the broad ligament to the pelvic lymph nodes.** In advanced-stage disease, there may be retrograde dissemination via the lymphatics of this pathway to **the round ligament to the inguinal lymph nodes.**
  - The second follows **the ovarian vein to the paracaval and paraaortic** lymph nodes, particularly in advanced-stage disease.

- Spread through the lymphatic channels of the diaphragm and through the retroperitoneal lymph nodes can lead to dissemination above the diaphragm, especially to **the left supraclavicular lymph nodes & its enlargement,** due to obstruction of the efferent lymphatic channel of the nodes by the tumor emboli, as it enters the thoracic duct just prior to its drainage into the left subclavian vein.

3. HEMATOGENOUS

- Hematogenous dissemination at the time of diagnosis is **uncommon**. Spread to the lungs and liver parenchyma, occurs in only 2-3% of patients. Most patients when diagnosed have a **right pleural effusion**. Systemic metastases are frequent who have survived for some years and particularly in poorly differentiated tumors refractory to combination chemotherapy.

4. DIRECT

- After the capsule is broken, the spread occurs directly to the adjacent organs such as tubes, broad ligament, intestines, omentum & uterus.

PROGNOSTIC FACTORS

PATHOLOGIC FACTORS

- **Histologic type** (**clear cell carcinomas** are associated with worse prognosis than that of other histologic types).

- **Histologic grade** (determined either by the pattern of differentiation or by the **extent of cellular anaplasia and the proportion of undifferentiated cells**). However, Grading of ovarian cancers is having high degree of intraobserver and interobserver variation.

BIOLOGIC FACTORS

- Determining ploidy using flow cytometry. There is a high correlation between **FIGO stage and ploidy;** low-stage cancers tend to be diploid and high-stage tumors tend to be aneuploid. So, ploidy is an independent prognostic variable and one of the most significant predictors of survival.

- Flow cytometric analysis also provides data on the **cell cycle,** and the proliferation fraction (S phase) determined by this technique has correlated with prognosis.

- Out of more than 100 **proto-oncogenes** HER-2/neu oncogene is expressed by **30% of epithelial ovarian tumors** & has poorer prognosis, especially patients who have more than 5 copies of the gene.

- **The most commonly expressed tumor suppressor gene in ovarian cancer is p53.** Indeed, 50% of all epithelial ovarian cancers have evidence of mutated p53. Other tumor suppressor genes that are being evaluated are **ras and PTEN.**

- A significant inverse correlation has been reported between **clonogenic growth in vitro** and survival. Multivariate analysis has found that clonogenic growth in a semisolid culture medium is a significant independent prognostic variable. The use of an extreme drug resistance assay has been suggested as a possible means of directing therapy by defining platinum-sensitive and resistant tumors in vitro.

CLINICAL FACTORS

- In addition to stage, **the extent of residual disease after primary surgery, the volume of ascites and patient's age and performance status** are all independent prognostic variables.

- Among patients with stage I disease, **tumor grade, capsular penetration, surface excrescences, malignant ascites and dense adherence to the pelvic peritoneum** had a significant adverse impact on prognosis, whereas intraoperative tumor spillage or rupture did not rather tumors found to have already ruptured preoperatively do have a poorer prognosis.

PREVENTION

(1) Parity $\propto$ 1/the risk of ovarian cancer, having at least one child is protective of the disease, **with a risk reduction of 0.3 to 0.4.**

(2) **OCP use ↓ses risk** approx. 10% per year to 50% after 5 years of use by…↓se in menstrual blood loss and therefore with ↓sed retrograde menstruation.

- <u>OCP is the only documented method of chemoprevention for ovarian cancer.</u> It is important for women with a strong family history of ovarian cancer.

(3) **Fenretinide (4-hydroxyretinoic acid)**, a vitamin A derivative, has been given to women with unilateral breast cancer in an effort to reduce the risk of contralateral breast cancer. Trials are going to determine its role in prevention of ovarian cancer.

(4) **Prophylactic salpingo-oophorectomy (the most effective)** reduces, but does not eliminate, the risk of ovarian and fallopian tube cancers. Because the entire peritoneum is at risk, peritoneal carcinomas can occur in 2-3% of women even after prophylactic BSO. The ovaries may provide protection from cardiovascular and orthopedic diseases, and long-term mortality may not be decreased by the performance of prophylactic oophorectomy particularly in premenopausal women who don't have any risk factors for ovarian cancer.

MANAGEMENT OF EPITHELIAL OVARIAN CANCER

- In select patients, minimally invasive procedures may be used for surgical staging. (N15)

- In early-stage disease, minimally invasive techniques to achieve the surgical goals may be considered in selected patients. (N15)

PRIMARY TREATMENT

NEOADJUVANT CHEMOTHERAPY

- Benefit of neoadjuvant chemotherapy f/b interval cytoreduction remains controversial.

- May be considered for patients with bulky stage III to IV disease who are not surgical candidates. This assessment should be made before neoadjuvant chemotherapy is administered.

- Standard IV regimens described in the algorithm may be used for neoadjuvant chemotherapy.

- More data is necessary prior to recommending neoadjuvant chemotherapy in potentially resectable ovarian cancer, and upfront debulking surgery remains the treatment of choice in the US. (N15)

- A randomized phase III trial assessed neoadjuvant chemotherapy with interval debulking surgery versus upfront primary debulking surgery in extensive-stage IIIC/IV ovarian, primary peritoneal, and Fallopian tube carcinoma (sponsored by the EORTC-GCG and the NCIC-CTG). Median overall survival was equivalent in these patients, but patients receiving neoadjuvant chemotherapy with interval debulking surgery had fewer complications.

- A major criticism of this international trial is that reported PFS and overall survival were inferior to those reported more recently in randomized studies in the US of patients undergoing primary debulking f/b postop IV chemotherapy for advanced ovarian cancer. Although the median overall survival in the international trial is 20 months lower than that reported in U.S. trials using the primary debulking f/b chemotherapy, this difference may have been a result of selection of patients at higher risk to the international trial (which did not include stage IIIB or earlier-stage cancer). Also, primary or interval debulking surgery in the international trial may have been suboptimal (i.e., patients may have had >1 cm of residual disease).

- A recent retrospective analysis of the EORTC-NCIC trial reported that stage IV disease had longer survival with neoadjuvant therapy, whereas stage IIIC disease and less bulky tumors had longer survival with upfront surgery.

SURGICAL STAGING FOR EARLY STAGE & PRIMARY CYTOREDUCTIVE SURGERY FOR ADVANCED STAGE

- Already mentioned.

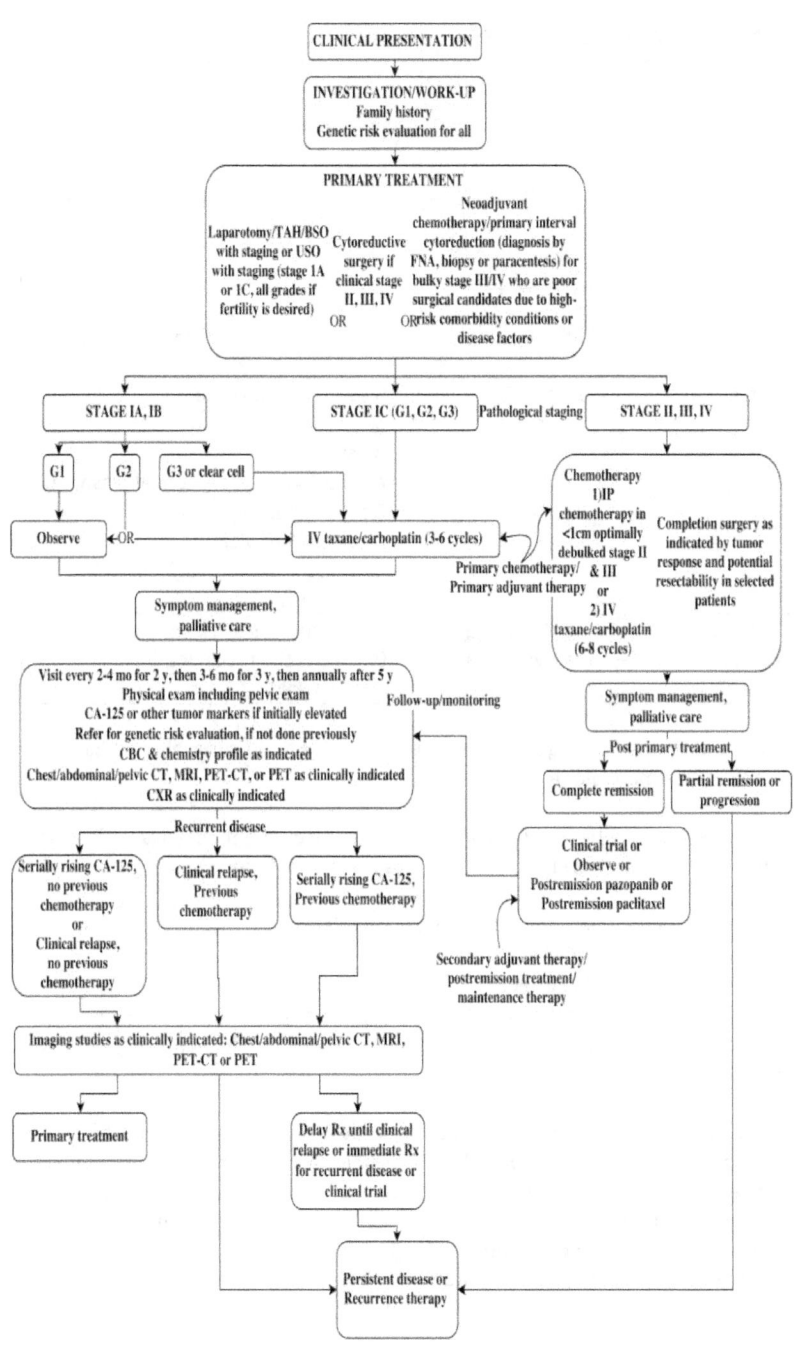

POST OPERATIVE CHEMOTHERAPY/PRIMARY CHEMOTHERAPY/ADJUVANT CHEMOTHERAPY

- Most patients with epithelial ovarian cancer receive postoperative systemic chemotherapy.

EARLY-STAGE EPITHELIAL OVARIAN CANCER RISK GROUPS	
Low Risk	**High Risk**
- Stage IA or IB, grade 1 and 2	- Stage IA or IB, grade 3 - Stage IC - All stage II - Ascites/positive peritoneal washing - Dense adherence - Clear-cell histology - Tumor on external surface - Capsule rupture
- The standard treatment is surgery alone, and the 5-year survival is at least 95%.	- This group has a relapse risk of 40-50% and is the focus of adjuvant therapy trials.

- Observation is for stage IA or IB, G1 tumors, because survival is >90% with surgical treatment alone.

- Taxanes should be included in the primary treatment of advanced-stage epithelial ovarian cancer, unless there **are contraindications.**

- 2nd generation platinum analogue, carboplatin has less toxicity than its parent compound, cisplatin.
   - Fewer GI side effects, especially nausea and vomiting,
   - Less nephrotoxicity, neurotoxicity, and ototoxicity.

Carboplatin is, however, associated with a higher degree of myelosuppression.

- **The dose of carboplatin is calculated by using the AUC and the GFR according to the Calvert formula. The target AUC is 5 to 6 for previously untreated patients with ovarian cancer. Alternatively, a dose of approximately 350-450 mg/m^2 carboplatin can be used initially in patients with a normal serum creatinine and adjusted to toxicity. A platelet nadir of approximately 50,000/mL is a suitable target.**

- The intravenous/IP chemotherapy regimen (IP chemotherapy) is recommended for stage III with optimally debulked (<1 cm residual) disease based on RCTs (category 1). Stage II may also receive IP chemotherapy, although no randomized evidence for stage II has been published.

- Who are not candidates for IP therapy (e.g., those with poor performance status), other regimens may be recommended. IV docetaxel plus carboplatin (category 1) (for who are at high risk for neuropathy e.g., diabetes) or paclitaxel plus cisplatin (category 1) are options for alternative regimens. Number of cycles of treatment varies with the stage.

- Some feel there is a survival advantage for 6 cycles of chemotherapy in patients with serous cytology.

- IV regimens:
- Paclitaxel, 175 mg/m^2 over 3-hr IV infusion, f/b carboplatin, dosed at an AUC of 5 to 6 IV over 1 hr on day 1, given every 3 weeks for 6 cycles (category 1) (sensory peripheral neuropathy)
- Dose-dense paclitaxel, 80 mg/m^2 IV over 1 hr on days 1, 8, and 15 plus carboplatin AUC 5 to 6 IV over 1 hr on day 1, every 3 weeks for 6 cycles (category 1) (increased anemia and decreased quality of life) better PFS and overall survival but toxic
- Paclitaxel 60 mg/m^2 over 1 hr f/b carboplatin AUC 2 IV over 30 minutes, weekly for 18 weeks (category 1) (fewer side effects & better quality of life) for elderly or those with poor performance status (sensory peripheral neuropathy) and
- Docetaxel, 60-75 mg/m^2 1-hr IV infusion f/b carboplatin, dosed at AUC of 5 to 6 intravenous over 1 hr on day 1, every 3 weeks for 6 cycles (category 1). **the docetaxel has fewer neurologic effects, arthralgias, myalgias, and extremity weakness** than the paclitaxel. However, **the docetaxel plus carboplatin regimen is associated with significantly more myelosuppression and its consequences, i.e., serious infections and prolonged grade 3-4 neutropenia.**

Note: These IV regimens may also be used for neoadjuvant chemotherapy

- IP regimen:
- Paclitaxel, 135 mg/m^2 continuous IV infusion over 3 or 24 hours on day 1; cisplatin, 75-100 mg/m^2 IP on day 2 after IV paclitaxel; paclitaxel, 60 mg/m^2 IP on day 8; repeat every 3 weeks for 6 cycles (category 1) (leucopenia, infection, fatigue, renal toxicity, abdominal discomfort, and neurotoxicity). Note that these IP regimens include IV regimens so that systemic disease can also be treated. (A 3-hour infusion of paclitaxel has not been proven to be equivalent to a 24-hour infusion, although a 3-hour infusion has been reported to be more convenient, easier to tolerate, and less toxic. Many centers

modified the dose of cisplatin to 75 mg/m^2 rather than 100 mg/m^2 to reduce toxicity. Others substitute carboplatin (AUC 6) for cisplatin in the regimen).

- Whether to use IP or intravenous chemotherapy remains controversial.

- Note that there are no agents to prevent chemotherapy-induced peripheral neuropathy.

- Patients considered for the IP cisplatin and IP/intravenous paclitaxel regimen should have normal renal function before starting, a medically appropriate PS based on the future toxicities of the IP/intravenous regimen, and no previous evidence of medical problems that could significantly worsen during chemotherapy (e.g., preexisting neuropathy)

- Reasons for discontinuing the IP regimen included catheter complications, nausea, vomiting, dehydration, and abdominal pain. Women unable to complete IP therapy should receive intravenous therapy. Techniques to decrease catheter complications include catheter choice and timing of insertion. Giving intravenous hydration before and after IP chemotherapy is a useful strategy to prevent renal toxicity. After chemotherapy, patients often require IV fluids (5-7 days) in the outpatient setting to prevent or help treat dehydration.

- Patients with poor PS, comorbidities, stage IV disease, or advanced age (>65 years) may not tolerate the IP regimen or the other combination IV regimens described in the NCCN Guidelines. Single-agent platinum agents, such as cisplatin or carboplatin, may be more appropriate for these patients.

- All women should be counseled about the clinical benefit associated with combined intravenous and IP chemotherapy administration before undergoing surgery for epithelial ovarian cancer, Fallopian tube cancer, primary peritoneal cancer, or MMMT.

- Median PFS was significantly increased without increase in overall survival and/or improved quality of life in patients receiving prolonged bevacizumab (upfront with carboplatin/paclitaxel and as maintenance therapy) when compared with chemotherapy alone in 2 phase III randomized trials (GOG 0218, ICON7). NCCN recommends (category 3) that if bevacizumab is used with upfront chemotherapy followed by maintenance therapy, then either the GOG 0218 or ICON7 regimens should be used. **Bevacizumab 7.5-15 mg/kg** can be added to any of IV or IP chemotherapy regimen containing carboplatin & paclitaxel.

- There is no evidence that >6-8 cycles of combination chemotherapy are required for initial (neoadjuvant + primary adjuvant) chemotherapy for patients with stage II to IV disease. They may receive 3-6 cycles of neoadjuvant chemotherapy f/b completion surgery & primary adjuvant chemotherapy.

RECOMMENDATIONS AFTER PRIMARY TREATMENT

- After initial treatment (e.g., 6 cycles of chemotherapy), patients should undergo a clinical re-evaluation...
  - Who have complete clinical remission observation with follow-up is recommended,
  - Who have partial remission or progression during initial treatment should be treated with second-line approaches (see persistent or recurrent disease).

MAINTENANCE THERAPY/SECONDARY ADJUVANT THERAPY/ POSTREMISSION TREATMENT

- Options for maintenance therapy for the management of advanced-stage (stages II–IV) disease who are in complete clinical remission after their initial therapeutic regimen include...
  - Observation alone,
  - A clinical trial, or
  - Additional systemic therapy increases PFS
    - **Pazopanib** [category 2B], FDA not approved, not increases overall survival, increases risk of grade 3 or 4 hypertension
    - **Paclitaxel** [category 3], 135-175 mg/m^2 every 4 weeks for 12 cycles, increases toxicity
    - **Bevacizumab** [category 3] increases PFS when administered following initial chemotherapy that included bevacizumab. No data to support introducing bevacizumab as maintenance therapy if other initial primary regimens were used

- Complete clinical remission is defined as no objective evidence of disease (i.e., negative physical examination, negative CA-125 levels, negative CT with <1 cm lymph nodes).

- Topotecan, cisplatin, IV OvaRex/oregovomab (anti-CA125), IP yttrium-labeled antimucin HMFG (human milk fat globulin) MonAb failed to show any benefits as maintenance therapy.

FOLLOW-UP/MONITORING

- Follow-up is required after complete clinical remission to monitor for recurrent disease.

- Patients should be educated about the signs and symptoms suggestive of recurrence (e.g., pelvic pain, bloating, early satiety, obstruction, weight loss, fatigue).

- Who have had fertility-sparing surgery should be monitored by ultrasound examinations if necessary; completion surgery should be considered (category 2B) after they finish childbearing.

- If CA-125 was initially elevated, the measurement of a CA-125 level or other tumor markers is recommended. SGO states that use of CA-125 levels for surveillance is optional. The NCCN recommends that patients should discuss the pros & cons of CA-125 monitoring.

MANAGEMENT OF AN INCREASING CA-125 LEVEL

- Patients who are found to have an increasing CA-125 level during routine monitoring and follow-up but no signs or symptoms of recurrent disease, following an evaluation with imaging techniques & examination includes...
- Who have never received chemotherapy should be managed using recommendations for newly diagnosed patients, should undergo clinically appropriate imaging studies and surgical debulking, and should be treated as previously described (see Primary Treatment).
- Who have received chemotherapy should be managed with...
  - Recurrence therapy (drugs, radiation, or other treatment to decrease tumor burden, control symptoms, or increase length and/or quality of life).
  - Observation until clinical symptom arises. After the documentation of an increased CA-125 level (i.e., biochemical relapse), the median time for a clinical relapse is 2 to 6 months. Immediate treatment for biochemical relapse is not beneficial.
  - Enrollment in a clinical trial. Because tamoxifen and other hormonally active agents have a defined response rate for patients with recurrent disease who have progressed after platinum-based chemotherapy, these agents are frequently administered to patients who have only a rising CA-125 level as evidence of tumor progression.

MANAGEMENT OF RECURRENT DISEASE

TYPES	RELAPSE	On subsequent chemotherapy	
		Response rate	Median survival
Platinum sensitive	6 months or more after primary chemotherapy	27-65%	12-24 mo
Platinum resistant	Within 6 months of primary chemotherapy	10-30%	6-9 mo
Platinum refractory	Progresses after 2 consecutive chemotherapy regimens without ever sustaining a clinical benefit. Progression is defined using RECIST (Response Evaluation Criteria in Solid Tumor) criteria	<10%	3-5 mo

- The goals of treatment include...
- **Improving control of disease related symptoms,**
- **Maintaining or improving quality of life,**
- **Delaying time to progression and**
- **Prolonging survival (particularly in women with platinum-sensitive recurrences).**

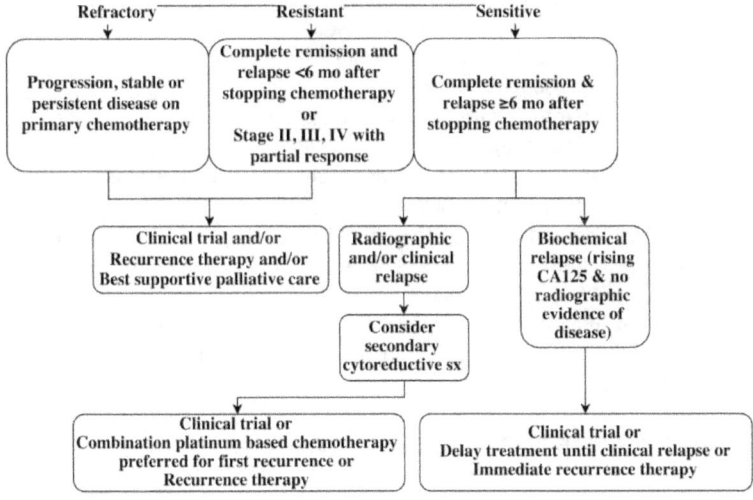

- Before any drug is given in the recurrent setting, patient should be an appropriate candidate for the drug (e.g., adequate renal or hepatic function). Patients receiving multiple sequential courses of chemotherapy may experience excessive toxicity and may not be able to tolerate doses used for first-line recurrence therapy; thus, clinical judgment should be used when selecting doses.

- **Recurrence therapy** refers to therapy (e.g., drugs, radiation, or other treatment) that is given for recurrent cancer to control symptoms and increase length or quality of life for clinical, biochemical, or radiographic evidence of recurrent cancer following initial treatment.

PLATINUM-SENSITIVE

- The longer the interval of relapse, the higher the probability of a secondary response to secondary platinum-based chemotherapy.

- Studies show advantage of a second line regimen containing both paclitaxel and a platinum agent compared with platinum-based therapy alone in patients who have not received paclitaxel in their primary chemotherapeutic regimen.

- For platinum-sensitive recurrence options are... (N15)
- Platinum-based combination chemotherapy is recommended (category 1)
    o Carboplatin/paclitaxel
    o Carboplatin/liposomal doxorubicin (superior PFS to carboplatin/paclitaxel, but easier to tolerate with less severe toxicities, widely used)
    o Carboplatin/weekly paclitaxel,
    o Carboplatin/docetaxel,
    o Carboplatin/gemcitabine (improves PFS),
    o Cisplatin/gemcitabine.
- Who cannot tolerate combination therapy, the preferred single agent is carboplatin or cisplatin,
- Carboplatin/gemcitabine/bevacizumab for who have not previously received bevacizumab (2B). Bevacizumab combination regimens improve PFS (OCEANS trial),
- Bevacizumab alone (especially those with ascites) (2A) (hypertension, arterial thrombosis, or intestinal perforation),
- Olaparib.

PLATINUM RESISTANT- REFRACTORY

- Platinum-resistant disease requires the use of non-cross-resistant agents. Single-agent therapy is typically used, because combination regimens are associated with more toxicity without additional benefit. (N12)

- Some have used non-platinum drugs to prolong the "platinum-free interval", hoping that their use will allow the tumor to become platinum sensitive during the interval use of non-cross-resistant agents (not proved). (N12)

- For platinum-resistant disease non-platinum based options are... (N15)
- Docetaxel, oral etoposide, gemcitabine, liposomal doxorubicin, weekly paclitaxel, topotecan; sequential therapy using single agents is typically used.
- Weekly paclitaxel/bevacizumab, liposomal doxorubicin/bevacizumab, topotecan/bevacizumab. Bevacizumab combination regimens improve PFS & overall survival (AURELIA trial) but contraindicated in patients at increased risk of GI perforation or those who have previously received bevacizumab.
- Bevacizumab alone (especially those with ascites) (2A),
- Olaparib.

- **PACLITAXEL** It is fatigue and peripheral neuropathy.

- **DOCETAXEL** It is complicated by severe neutropenia.

- TOPOTECAN
Active second line treatment for patients with platinum sensitive and platinum resistant disease.
- $2.0 \ mg/m^2/d$ for 3 days every 3 week
- $1.5 \ mg/m^2/d$ for 5 days every 3 week
- $1.0 \ mg/m^2/d$ for 3 days every 3 week (similar response with lower toxicity)
- Continuous infusion $0.4 \ mg/m^2/d$ for 14 to 21 days
- $4 \ mg/m^2$/week for 3 weeks with a week off every month produce a response rate similar to the 5 day regimen with less toxicity & is preferred dose schedule in the recurrent setting.

Toxicity of topotecan is hematologic especially neutropenia.
Oral topotecan ($2.3 \ mg/m^2/d$ for 5 days every 3 weeks) produces results in similar response rates with less hematologic toxicity.

- LIPOSOMAL DOXORUBICIN
The most important side effect is the hand-foot syndrome (palmer-planter erythrodysesthesia or acral erythema) which occurs in 20% of patients who receive $50 \ mg/m^2$ every 4 weeks.
It is preferred to give $40 \ mg/m^2$ and escalate only if there are no side effects.

- GEMCITABINE
Myelosuppression and gastrointestinal.

- ETOPSIDE
Myelosuppression (grade 4 neutropenia) and gastrointestinal (nausea, vomiting).

- However, regardless of which regimen is selected initially, reevaluation should follow after 2 to 4 cycles of chemotherapy to determine if patients benefited from chemotherapy.

- Patients who primarily progress on 2 consecutive chemotherapy regimens without evidence of clinical benefit may not benefit from additional therapy.

OTHER POTENTIALLY ACTIVE AGENTS

- Cytotoxic substances like altretamine, capecitabine, cyclophosphamide, doxorubicin, ifosfamide, irinotecan, melphalan, oxaliplatin, paclitaxel, nanoparticle albumin-bound paclitaxel (i.e., nab-paclitaxel), pemetrexed, and vinorelbine,
- Hormonal therapies with tamoxifen, aromatase inhibitors (exemestane, anastrozole, letrozole), leuprolide acetate, or megestrol acetate are options for patients who cannot tolerate or have not responded to cytotoxic regimens,
- Palliative localized radiation therapy (development of acute & chronic intestinal morbidity, avoided). Patients who receive radiation are prone to vaginal stenosis, which can impair sexual function. Women can use vaginal dilators to prevent or treat vaginal stenosis. Dilator use can start 2 to 4 weeks after RT is completed and can be done indefinitely.

- Olaparib (AZD2281)...
  - PARP (poly ADP-ribose polymerase) inhibitor,
  - Active in select patients (those with BRCA1 and BRCA2 mutations have higher response rates than those who are BRCA negative) with chemotherapy-refractory ovarian cancer, especially those with platinum-sensitive disease,
  - Platinum resistant or refractory have a lower response rate to olaparib,
  - FDA & NCCN approved olaparib for patients with advanced ovarian cancer who have received treatment with 3 or more lines of chemotherapy and who have a germline BRCA mutation.
  - Not recommended by NCCN as maintenance therapy for patients with platinum-sensitive disease.

TARGETED THERAPIES

- Knowledge of molecular pathways within normal and malignant cells is leading to the development of cancer treatment agents with specific molecular targets.

- Under investigation. None has yet been approved.

- Genes within the PI3K/AKT and MAP kinase pathways have commanded the most attention based on early molecular investigations. For example,

- Potential druggable targets for **clear cell carcinoma of the ovary include mTOR, PI3K, c-MET, and VEGF.**
- Low-grade serous carcinomas have a 5% frequency of BRAF mutations and a 20% to 40% frequency of KRAS mutations, the MAP kinase pathway is a major focus for therapeutics. In the initial phase II trial of the **MEK inhibitor, selumetinib, for recurrent low-grade serous carcinoma**, a promising response rate of 15% was observed.

- Other novel agents under investigation include **antifolate receptor antibodies, vaccines, various immunologic therapies, and drugs that may affect p53-mutated cancer cells**, among others.

- There is a great potential in targeting angiogenesis, in particular VEGF, which plays a major role in the biology of EOC...

- The 1st target is to target VEGF itself (bevacizumab),
- The 2nd to target the VEGF receptor (VEGF Trap in phase II trials),
- The 3rd is to inhibit tyrosine kinase activation and downstream signaling with small molecules that work at the cellular level (in clinical trials).

- Bevacizumab is humanized monoclonal antibody that targets angiogenesis by binding to VEGF-A, thereby blocking the interaction of VEGF with its receptor.

The response rates in both platinum sensitive and refractory patients range from 16-22%.

The side effects include hypertension (MC), fatigue, proteinuria, gastrointestinal perforation/fistula (most concerning), vascular thrombosis, CNS ischemia, pulmonary hypertension, bleeding, and wound healing complications.

The bowel perforation complication can be avoided by carefully screening patient by limiting bevacizumab treatment to patients without...

- Clinical symptoms of bowel obstruction,
- Evidence of rectosigmoid involvement on pelvic examination,
- Bowel involvement on CT scan.

- VEGF trap functions as a soluble decoy receptor soaking up ligand before it can interact with its receptor.

MANAGEMENT OF WOMEN AT HIGH RISK FOR OVARIAN CANCER

FAMILY HISTORY (see risk factors)

- The management must be individualized and **depends on her age, her reproductive plans, and the extent of risk.** In all of these syndromes, women at risk benefit from a thorough **pedigree analysis.**

PEDIGREE ANALYSIS (BOTH MATERNAL & PATERNAL SIDES OF THE FAMILY)

- The risk of carrying a germline mutation that predisposes to ovarian cancer **depends on the number of first- and/or second-degree relatives (or both) with a history of epithelial ovarian carcinoma or breast cancer (or both), and on the number of malignancies that occur at an earlier age.**

- A geneticist should evaluate the family pedigree for **at least three generations.** Decisions about management are best made after careful study and, whenever possible, verification of the histologic diagnosis of the family members' ovarian cancer.

- In families with **two first-degree relatives (i.e., mother, sister, or daughter) with documented premenopausal epithelial ovarian cancer**, the risk that a female first-degree relative has an affected gene could be as high as 35-40%.

- In families with a **single first-degree relative and a single second-degree relative (i.e., grandmother, aunt, first cousin, or granddaughter) with epithelial ovarian cancer,** the risk that a woman has an affected gene also may be increased. The risk may be 2 to 10 fold higher than in those without a familial history of the disease.

- In families with a **single postmenopausal first-degree relative with epithelial ovarian carcinoma**, a woman may not have an increased risk of having an affected gene because the case is most likely to be sporadic. However, **if the ovarian cancer occurs in a premenopausal relative**, this could be significant, and a full pedigree analysis should be undertaken.

- Women with a **primary history of breast cancer** have twice the expected incidence of subsequent ovarian cancer.

ADD PREVENTION

RECOMMENDATIONS

- <u>Women at high risk for ovarian or breast cancer</u> should undergo **genetic counseling** and, if the risk appears to be substantial, may be offered **genetic testing for BRCA1 and BRCA2.**

- <u>Who wish to preserve their reproductive capacity</u> can undergo **screening by TVS every 6 months.**

- **OCP should be recommended** to young women before they embark on an attempt to have a family.

- <u>Women who do not wish to maintain their fertility or who have completed their families</u> should be recommended to undergo **prophylactic BSO after 35 years, but by 40 year.** The risk of ovarian cancers under 40 is very low but the decision regarding the age of surgery should be based on the age of onset of ovarian cancers in the family. Most BRCA-2 related ovarian cancers tend to occur after 50, whereas BRCA-1 related cancers occur at an earlier age. The risk should be clearly documented, preferably established by BRCA1 and BRCA2 testing, before oophorectomy is performed. Prophylactic salpingo-oophorectomy...

- **Reduces the risk of BRCA-related gynecologic cancer by 96%.**
- Reduces the risk of developing subsequent **breast cancer by 50-80%.**
- Although the risk of ovarian cancer is significantly diminished, there remains the small risk of **primary peritoneal carcinoma,** a tumor for which women who have mutations in BRCA1 and BRCA2 may have a higher predisposition. The risk of subsequent development of peritoneal carcinoma is **0.8-1 %.**
- They have a **risk of harboring occult neoplasia.**

Risk-Reducing Salpingo-Oophorectomy (RRSO) Protocol (BRCA/HBOC syndrome) (N15)

- Perform operative laparoscopy.
- Survey upper abdomen, bowel surfaces, omentum, appendix (if present), and pelvic organs.
- Biopsy any abnormal peritoneal findings.
- Obtain pelvic washing for cytology. (50 cc NS instilled and aspirated immediately)
- Perform total BSO, removing 2 cm of proximal ovarian vasculature/IP ligament, all tube up to the cornua, and all peritoneum surrounding the ovaries and tubes, especially peritoneum underlying areas of adhesion between tube and/or ovary and the pelvic sidewall.
- Engage in minimal instrument handling of the tubes and ovaries to avoid traumatic exfoliation of cells.

- Both ovaries and tubes should be placed in an endobag for retrieval from the pelvis.
- Both ovaries and tubes should be processed according to SEE-FIM protocol.
- If occult malignancy or STIC (serous tubal intraepithelial carcinoma) identified, provide referral to gynecologic oncologist.

Principle: Fallopian tube may be the origin of serous ovarian and primary peritoneal cancers, including serous intraepithelial carcinoma of the Fallopian tube (also known as STIC).

- <u>In women who also have a strong family history of breast or ovarian cancer,</u> **annual breast screening using a combination of MRI, mammograms, and ultrasound should be performed beginning at age 30 years.**

- <u>Women with a documented HNPCC syndrome</u> should be treated as above, but in addition, they should undergo **periodic colonoscopy, endometrial biopsy, or prophylactic hysterectomy after the completion of childbearing.**

PROPHYLACTIC HYSTERECTOMY IN HIGH-RISK WOMEN

- **Controversial.** Although most studies show no increase in the rate of uterine and cervical tumors, there are some reports of **an increase of papillary serous tumors of the endometrium.**

- Women on **tamoxifen are at higher risk for benign endometrial lesions (e.g., polyps) and endometrial cancer.** Therefore, it is reasonable to consider the performance of a **prophylactic hysterectomy in conjunction with salpingo-oophorectomy,** and this decision should be individualized.

PROGNOSIS

- The **survival** of women **who have a BRCA1 or BRCA2 mutation and develop ovarian cancer is longer** than that for those who do not have a mutation.

OVARIAN LOW MALIGNANT POTENTIAL (LMP) TUMORS (BORDERLINE EPITHELIAL OVARIAN TUMORS) (BORDERLINE OVARIAN TUMOR) (ATYPICAL PROLIFERATIVE TUMOR)

- Ovarian LMP tumor is typically serous (see serous borderline epithelial ovarian tumor); other histologic subtypes can also occur.

- LMP is a primary epithelial ovarian lesion with cytologic characteristics suggesting malignancy but without frank invasion and with a clinically indolent course and good prognosis.

- Five-year survival exceeds 80%.

- In contrast to patients with frankly invasive ovarian carcinoma, women with ovarian LMP tumors tend to be younger, are often diagnosed with stage I disease, and are candidates for FSS.

- Pathologic hallmark of typical EOC is the identification of peritoneal implants, which microscopically and/or macroscopically invade the peritoneum. Ovarian LMP tumor has the visual appearance of peritoneal carcinomatosis. However, microscopic evaluation fails to reveal evidence of frank invasion by the tumor nodules, although rarely invasive implants (which continue to be consistent with the diagnosis of LMP lesions) can be identified microscopically by the pathologist.

PRIMARY TREATMENT

- Treatment guidelines depend on the histologic and clinical characteristics, the age of the patient, the stage of the disease at the time of diagnosis, and whether invasive implants are present.

- The principle treatment is surgical removal of primary tumor.

- If fertility is desired → USO at the time of comprehensive staging.

- If fertility not desired → observation or debulking surgery. However, data do not show increased survival with lymphadenectomy and omentectomy for LMP, although upstaging does occur.

- see flow chart.

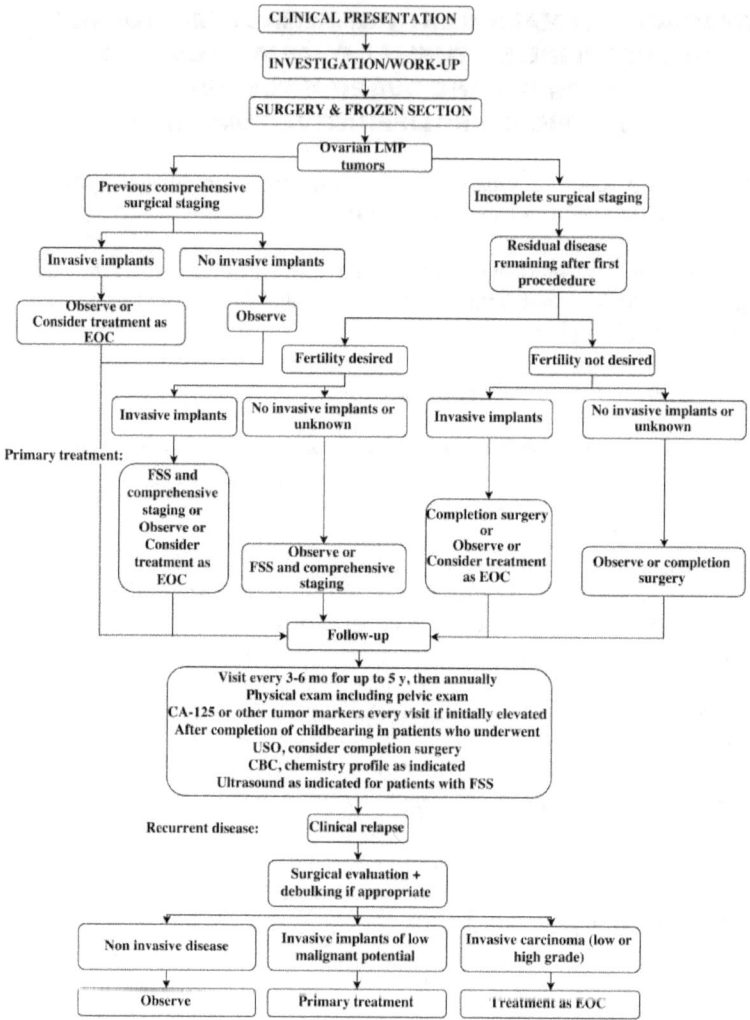

POST OPERATIVE CHEMOTHERAPY

- Invasive implants on the peritoneal surfaces in LMP tumors portend a less favorable prognosis; therefore, postoperative chemotherapy with the same regimens used for EOC can be considered. However, the **benefit of chemotherapy is controversial**. For patients who have no microscopically demonstrable invasive implants; observation is recommended.

FOLLOW-UP

- see flow chart.
- After childbearing is completed, completion surgery should be considered (2B).

RELAPSE

- Chances of recurrences are less and are associated with positive margins of the removed ovarian cyst.
- see flow chart.

SURVIVAL

Age	5 year survival
<50 years	40%
>50 years	15%

Stages	5 year survival
Stage I	94%
Stage II	73%
Stage III (IIIA-41%, IIIB-25%, IIIC-23%)	37%
Stage IV	25%

- Survival of patients with borderline tumors is excellent, with stage I lesions having a 98% 15-year survival. When all stages of borderline tumors are included, the 5-year survival rate is about 86-90%.
- For stage III disease...

At start of treatment	5-year survival
Microscopic residual disease	40-75%
Optimal cytoreduction	30-40%
Suboptimal cytoreduction	5%

- Patients whose **Karnofsky's index (KI) is low (<70) have a significantly shorter survival** than those with a KI >70.

GERM CELL MALIGNANCIES

INTRODUCTION/EPIDEMIOLOGY

- Their incidence is only about one tenth the incidence of malignant germ cell tumors of the testis.

- Although **20-25% of all benign and malignant ovarian neoplasms are of germ cell origin,** only about 3% of these are malignant.

- Germ cell malignancies account for **<5%** of all ovarian cancers in western countries; but **up to 15%** of ovarian cancers in Asian and African-American societies, where EOCs are much less common.

ORIGIN

- Arises from the **primordial (undifferentiated) germ cells of the ovary.**

- Can arise from **extragonadal sites (mediastinum and the retroperitoneum)** which is explained by the **embryonic migration of the germ cells from the caudal part of the yolk sac to the dorsal mesentery before their incorporation into the sex cords of the developing gonads.**

CLASSIFICATION

1. **Primitive germ cell tumors**
   - **A.** Dysgerminoma
   - **B.** Yolk sac tumor
   - **C.** Embryonal carcinoma
   - **D.** Polyembryoma
   - **E.** Non-gestational choriocarcinoma
   - **F.** Mixed germ cell tumor

2. **Bipashic or triphasic teratoma**
   - **A.** Immature teratoma
   - **B.** Mature teratoma [solid, cystic (dermoid cyst) & fetiform teratoma (homunuculus)]

3. **Monodermal teratoma and somatic-type tumors associated with dermoid cysts**
   - **A.** Thyroid tumor [Struma ovarii (benign, malignant)]
   - **B.** Carcinoid
   - **C.** Neuroectodermal
   - **D.** Carcinoma

E. Melanocytic
F. Sarcoma
G. Sebaceous tumor
H. Pituitary-type tumor
I. Retinal anlage tumor
J. Others (homunculus)

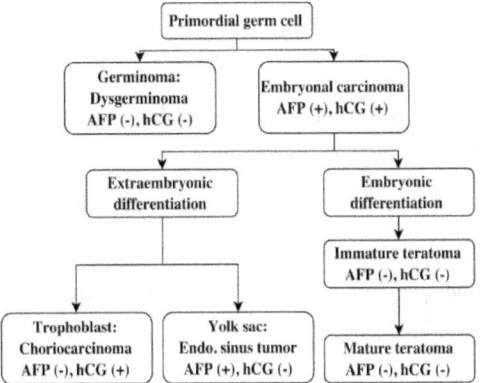

- Both **AFP and hCG** are secreted by some germ cell tumors & can be clinically useful in the diagnosis and in follow-up after surgery.

- **PLAP and LDH** are produced by up to 95% of dysgerminomas, and serial measurements of LDH may be useful for monitoring the disease.

- Embryonal carcinoma (a cancer composed of undifferentiated cells) synthesizes **both hCG and AFP,** and this lesion is the progenitor of several other germ cell tumors.

- More differentiated germ cell tumors, such as...
   • The endodermal sinus tumor, which secretes **AFP,** and
   • The choriocarcinoma, which secretes **hCG**
...are derived from the extraembryonic tissues.

- The **immature teratomas** derived **from the embryonic cells** have **lost the ability to secrete** these substances.

- Pure germinomas do not secrete these markers.

ETIOLOGY & RISK FACTORS

1) AGE:

- In the **first two decades** of life, ~**70% of ovarian tumors are of germ cell origin,** and 1/3rd of these are malignant. Germ cell cancers also are seen in the 3rd decade, but thereafter they become quite rare.

DYSGERMINOMA

- **MC malignant germ cell tumor,** accounting for ~**30-40% of all ovarian cancers of germ cell origin.**

- Represent only **1-3% of all ovarian cancers,** but **5-10% of all ovarian cancers in younger than 20 yr.**

- **75% of dysgerminomas** occur between **10-30 yr, 5% occur before 10 yr** & rarely occur after 50 yr.

- Because they occur in young, **20-30% of ovarian malignancies during pregnancy are dysgerminomas.**

- Found in both sexes and may arise in gonadal or extragonadal sites (**midline structures from the pineal gland to the mediastinum and the retroperitoneum).** Histologically, they represent abnormal proliferations of the basic germ cell. In the ovary, the germ cells are encapsulated at birth (the primordial follicle), and the unencapsulated or free cells die. If either of the latter processes fails, it is conceivable that the germ cell could free itself of its normal control and multiply indiscriminately.

- ~65% of dysgerminomas are stage I at diagnosis. ~85-90% of stage I tumors are confined to one ovary; **10-15% are bilateral.** In fact, **dysgerminoma is the only germ cell malignancy that has this significant rate of bilaterality.** Other germ cell tumors are rarely bilateral.

PATHOLOGY (N12)

GROSS

- The size varies widely (5-15 cm). The **capsule is slightly bosselated** and the consistency of the **cut surface is fleshy and pale tan to gray-brown in color.**

MICROSCOPIC

- **Large round, ovoid or polygonal cells** have **abundant, clear, very-pale-staining cytoplasm, large and irregular nuclei and prominent nucleoli. Mitotic figures** are usually numerous.

- The **arrangement of the elements are in lobules and nests separated by fibrous septa,** which are **extensively infiltrated with lymphocytes, plasma cells, granulomas with epithelioid cells and multinucleated giant cells.**

- When necrosis is extensive, the lesion may be confused with **tuberculosis.**

- Occasional dysgerminomas **may contain syncytiotrophoblastic giant cells** and may be associated with **precocious puberty or virilization.**

- The presence of **calcifications** should prompt a search for a possible **underlying gonadoblastoma.**

- Dysgerminoma is a germ cell tumor and parthenogenesis (stimulation of the basic germ cell to atypical division) is the most commonly accepted genesis for the more immature teratomas, it is logical that these **two tumors may coexist. Choriocarcinoma, endodermal sinus tumor and other extraembryonal lesions are also commonly associated with the dysgerminoma.**

- ~**5% of dysgerminomas** are discovered in phenotypic women with abnormal gonads...
  - Pure gonadal dysgenesis (46, XY, bilateral streak gonads),
  - Mixed gonadal dysgenesis (45, X/46, XY, unilateral streak gonad, contralateral testis), and
  - The androgen insensitivity syndrome (46, XY, testicular feminization).

Therefore, for premenarcheal patients with a pelvic mass, the karyotype should be determined.

- For most patients with gonadal dysgenesis, dysgerminomas **arise in gonadoblastomas,** which are benign ovarian tumors that are composed of germ cells and sex cord stroma. If gonadoblastomas are left in situ in patients with gonadal dysgenesis, more than 50% will develop into ovarian malignancies.

- For patients whose contralateral ovary has been preserved, disease can develop in 5-10% of the retained gonads over the next 2 years. This figure includes those not given additional therapy, as well as patients with gonadal dysgenesis.

PATTERNS OF SPREAD (N12)

- 25% of patients who are diagnosed initially with metastatic disease, the tumor **most commonly spreads via the lymphatic system.** It can also **spread hematogenously or by direct extension** through the capsule of the ovary with exfoliation and dissemination of cells throughout the peritoneal surfaces.

- Metastases to the contralateral ovary may be present when there is no other evidence of spread.

- An uncommon site of metastatic disease is **bone (principally in lower vertebrae).**

- Metastases to the **lungs, liver, and brain** are seen in long-standing or recurrent disease. Metastasis to the **mediastinum and supraclavicular lymph nodes** is usually a late manifestation of disease.

PROGNOSIS (N12)

- If stage IA, USO alone results in a 5-year disease-free survival rate of greater than 95%.

- Recurrence chance increases in...
    - **Lesions >10-15 cm in diameter,**
    - **Age <20 years and**
    - **A microscopic pattern that includes numerous mitoses, anaplasia and a medullary pattern.**

- Surgery for advanced disease f/b chemotherapy with BEP or EC result in 5-yr survival rate of 85-90%.

IMMATURE TERATOMAS

- Contain elements that resemble tissues **derived from the embryo.**

- May occur **in combination with other germ cell tumors as mixed germ cell tumors.**

- Pure immature teratoma accounts for **<1% of all ovarian cancers,** but it is the **2nd MC germ cell malignancy.** Represent **10-20% of all ovarian malignancies seen in <20 years.**

- ~**50% of pure immature teratomas** occur in between **10-20 yr,** and rarely in postmenopausal women.

PATHOLOGY (N12)

- In the teratoma; recognition of the maturation of the various elements is important...
    - If maturation continues along normal lines, the mature or adult teratoma results, and the prognosis is excellent.
    - Conversely, abnormal maturation of these elements can result in an immature teratoma (rare) that has metastatic potential.
- Among the tumors with embryonal elements, those containing **neural tissues demonstrate most clearly the importance of the ability to mature.**

- Classified **based on the degree of differentiation & the quantity of immature tissue.** A determination of the **amount of undifferentiated (immature) neural tissue is of prognostic importance...**
    - Grade 1 is one in which <1 LPF contains immature neural elements,
    - Grade 2 has 1-3 LPFs with immature elements and
    - Grade 3 has >3 LPFs with immature elements.
- The significant inter- and intraobserver difficulty with a 3-tier system led to recommend the 2-tier grading system (**low grade or high grade**) in use.

- They may be associated with **gliomatosis peritonei,** a favorable prognostic finding if composed of completely mature tissues. These glial implants are not tumor derived but represent teratoma induced metaplasia of pluripotent mullerian stem cells in the peritoneum.

- Some of these lesions **contain calcifications similar to mature teratomas,** which can be detected by a radiograph of the abdomen or by ultrasonography. Rarely, they are associated with the **production of steroid hormones** and can be accompanied **by sexual pseudoprecocity.**

- Tumor markers are negative unless a mixed germ cell tumor is present.

PATTERNS OF SPREAD (N12)

- The MC **site is the peritoneum** and, much less common are the retroperitoneal lymph nodes. Blood borne metastases to organ parenchyma are uncommon & if present; seen in late or recurrent disease and in poorly differentiated tumors (i.e., grade 3).

PROGNOSIS (N12)

- Determined by the quantity of immature neural elements; with a **higher grade, there is a poorer prognosis.** This may not apply to children because they have a good outcome with surgery alone, regardless of the degree of immaturity.

- The **stage of disease** and the **extent of tumor at the initiation of treatment** have an impact on the curability of the lesion. Overall the 5-year survival rates for **all stages of pure immature teratoma is 70-80 %,** and it is **90-95% for patients with surgically staged, stage I lesions.**

- Somatic malignant change in benign cystic teratomas has been recorded in **0.5-2 % of cases,** usually in patients >40 yr. The **MC malignancy** developing **is squamous cell carcinoma.** Others are adenocarcinoma, melanomas (which may arise from skin or retinal anlage) & sarcomas (leiomyosarcomas & mixed mesodermal tumors). Carcinomas may arise from any of the epithelial elements. **Immature teratomas with malignant squamous elements** have a poorer prognosis.

ENDODERMAL SINUS TUMORS (YOLK SAC TUMORS)

- 3rd **MC malignant germ cell tumors** of the ovary.

- ESTs occur in patients with a **median age of 16-18 years**. About 1/3rd of the patients are premenarcheal at the time of diagnosis. (N12)

- Most patients have early-stage disease: 71%, stage I; 6%, stage II; and 23%, stage III. (N12)

PATHOLOGY (N12)

GROSS

- The gross appearance is **soft grayish-brown**. Cystic areas caused by degeneration in these rapidly growing lesions. The capsule is intact in most.

- **Unilateral in 100% of cases.**

MICROSCOPIC

- **Endodermal sinus or Schiller-Duval body**. The cystic space is lined with a layer of flattened or irregular endothelium into which projects a glomerulus like tuft with a central vascular core. These structures vary throughout the tumor, and the reticular, myxoid elements represent undifferentiated mesoblast. The lining of the papillary infolding and the cavity is irregular, with an occasional cell containing clear, glassy cytoplasm, simulating the hobnail appearance of the epithelium in clear cell tumors.

- Most EST lesions **secrete AFP** and, rarely **Alpha-1 antitrypsin**. AFP can be demonstrated in the tumor by means of the immunoperoxidase technique.

There is a good correlation between the extent of disease and the level of AFP, although discordance also has been observed.

- **Association of EST with gonadal dysgenesis must be appreciated,** and chromosomal analysis should be performed preoperatively in premenarcheal patients.

EMBRYONAL CARCINOMA

- An extremely rare tumor that is **distinguished from a choriocarcinoma of the ovary by the absence of syncytiotrophoblastic and cytotrophoblastic cells.**

- The patients are very young; ages ranged 4-28 yr. Older patients have been reported.

- **May secrete estrogens,** with the patient exhibiting **symptoms and signs of precocious pseudopuberty or irregular bleeding.**

- Clinical picture is otherwise **similar to that of the EST.** The primary **lesions tend to be large,** and about **two thirds are confined to one ovary** at the time of diagnosis.

- Secrete AFP and hCG.

CHORIOCARCINOMA OF THE OVARY

- Pure nongestational choriocarcinoma of the ovary is an extremely rare.

- Histologically, it has the **same appearance as gestational choriocarcinoma** metastatic to the ovaries.

- Most patients are <**20 yr.**

- **hCG can be useful in monitoring.** In the presence of high hCG levels, isosexual precocity has been seen to occur in about 50% whose lesions appear before menarche.

- Complete responses have been reported with **MAC (methotrexate, actinomycin D, and cyclophosphamide)** used in a manner described for GTDs. Alternatively, **BEP regimen** can be used.

- The prognosis is poor, with **most having metastases to organ parenchyma at the time of diagnosis.**

POLYEMBRYOMA

- Another extremely rare tumor, composed of embryoid bodies.

- This tumor replicates the **structures of early embryonic differentiation (i.e., the three somatic layers: endoderm, mesoderm, and ectoderm).**

- The lesion tends to occur in **very young, premenarcheal girls with signs of pseudopuberty and elevated AFP and hCG titers.**

- Anecdotally, the **VAC chemotherapeutic regimen** has been reported to be effective.

MIXED GERM CELL TUMORS

- Contain **two or more elements of the lesions** described above. The MC component is dysgerminoma (80%) f/b EST (70%) immature teratoma (53%) choriocarcinoma (20%) & embryonal carcinoma (16%).

- **Most frequent combination is a dysgerminoma and an EST.** The mixed lesions **may secrete either an AFP, hCG, or both or neither of these markers, depending on the components.**

- Should be managed with **BEP.** The serum marker, if positive initially, may become negative during chemotherapy, but this finding may reflect regression of only a particular component of the mixed lesion. Therefore, for these patients, **a second-look laparotomy** may be indicated to determine the precise response to therapy if macroscopic disease was present at initiation of chemotherapy.

- The **most important prognostic features are the size of the primary tumor and the relative size of its most malignant component.**

- For stage IA lesions <10 cm, survival is 100%. Tumors composed of **less than one third EST, choriocarcinoma, or grade 3 immature teratoma** also have an excellent prognosis, but it is less favorable when these components constitute most of the mixed lesions.

MANAGEMENT OF MALIGNANT GERM CELL TUMORS

- Workup may include...
  - Karyotyping in premenarcheal patients with pelvic mass,
  - PFTs if bleomycin is being considered.

PRIMARY TREATMENT

SURGICAL STAGING FOR EARLY STAGE & PRIMARY CYTOREDUCTIVE SURGERY FOR ADVANCED STAGE

- Basic principles already mentioned. Lymphadenectomy is important as dysgerminoma often metastasize to the para-aortic nodes around the renal vessels.

- After comprehensive complete surgical staging, observation is recommended for stage I dysgerminoma or immature teratoma. (N15)

- In children or adolescents with early-stage germ cell tumors, comprehensive staging may be omitted. If these patients have had incomplete surgical staging, recommended options depend on the type of tumor, the results of imaging and tumor marker (e.g., AFP, beta-HCG), age of the patient, and whether the patient desires fertility preservation. (N15)

- FSS (USO) if fertility desired, **regardless of stage** (because of the sensitivity of the tumor to chemotherapy) & should be monitored by ultrasound if necessary; completion surgery (category 2B) after finishing childbearing. (N15) If dysgerminoma is suspected and a small contralateral tumor is found, resect it and preserve some normal ovary. (N12)

- C/L ovarian involvement is rare with immature teratoma & 10-15 % in dysgerminoma. Routine resection or wedge biopsy of the C/L ovary is unnecessary; if suspicious mass then excisional biopsy is desirable. (N12)

- If karyotype reveals a Y chromosome, both ovaries should be removed, although the uterus may be left in situ for possible future embryo transfer. (N12)

- Immature teratomas are **much more chemosensitive. Cure depends on the ability to deliver chemotherapy promptly; so any surgical resection that may be morbid and therefore delay chemotherapy should be resisted.** (N12)

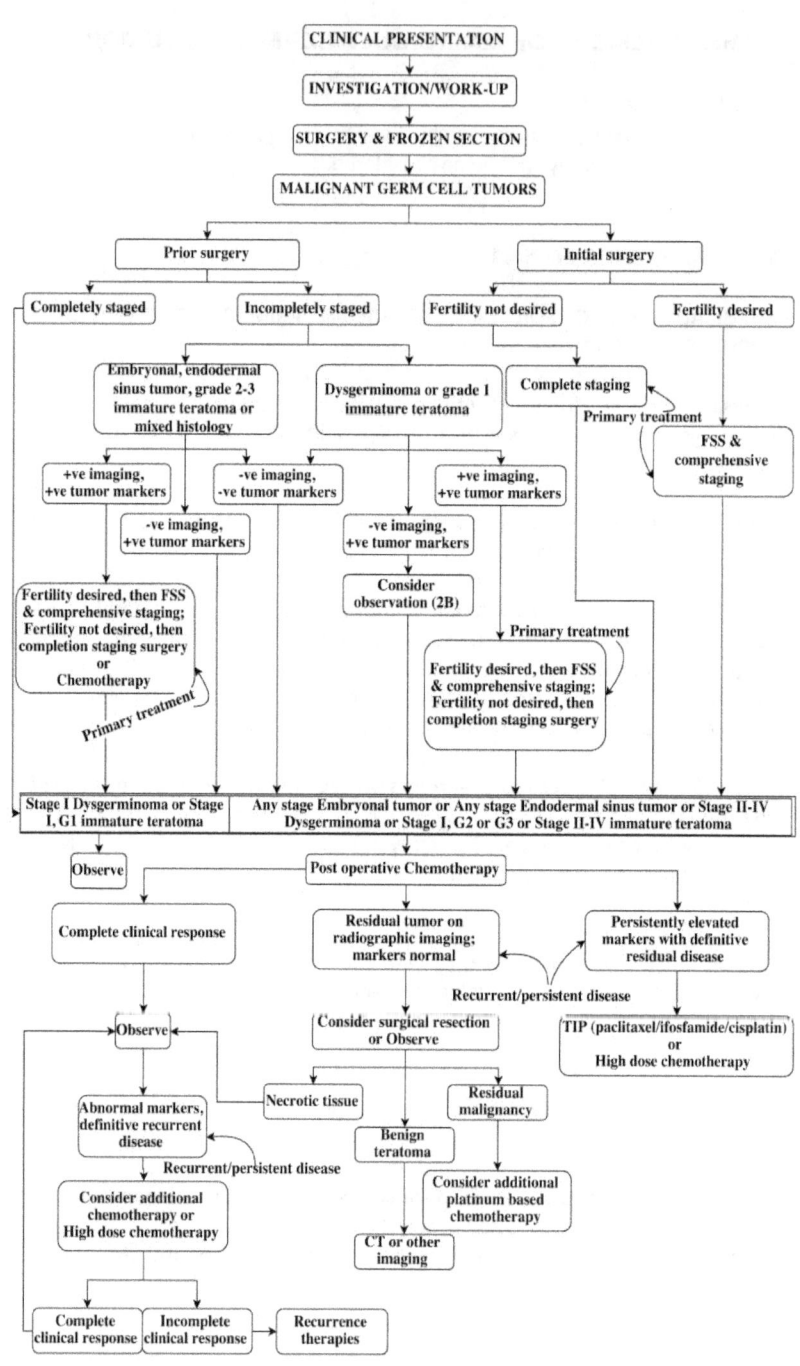

CLINICAL PRESENTATION

INVESTIGATION/WORK-UP

SURGERY & FROZEN SECTION

MALIGNANT GERM CELL TUMORS

Prior surgery

Initial surgery

Completely staged

Incompletely staged

Fertility not desired

Fertility desired

Embryonal, endodermal sinus tumor, grade 2-3 immature teratoma or mixed histology

Dysgerminoma or grade 1 immature teratoma

Complete staging

Primary treatment

FSS & comprehensive staging

+ve imaging, +ve tumor markers

-ve imaging, -ve tumor markers

+ve imaging, +ve tumor markers

-ve imaging, +ve tumor markers

-ve imaging, +ve tumor markers

Consider observation (2B)

Fertility desired, then FSS & comprehensive staging; Fertility not desired, then completion staging surgery or Chemotherapy

Primary treatment

Primary treatment

Fertility desired, then FSS & comprehensive staging; Fertility not desired, then completion staging surgery

Stage I Dysgerminoma or Stage I, G1 immature teratoma

Any stage Embryonal tumor or Any stage Endodermal sinus tumor or Stage II-IV Dysgerminoma or Stage I, G2 or G3 or Stage II-IV immature teratoma

Observe

Post operative Chemotherapy

Complete clinical response

Residual tumor on radiographic imaging; markers normal

Persistently elevated markers with definitive residual disease

Recurrent/persistent disease

Observe

Consider surgical resection or Observe

TIP (paclitaxel/ifosfamide/cisplatin) or High dose chemotherapy

Abnormal markers, definitive recurrent disease

Necrotic tissue

Residual malignancy

Benign teratoma

Recurrent/persistent disease

Consider additional chemotherapy or High dose chemotherapy

Consider additional platinum based chemotherapy

CT or other imaging

Complete clinical response

Incomplete clinical response

Recurrence therapies

POST OPERATIVE CHEMOTHERAPY/PRIMARY CHEMOTHERAPY/ADJUVANT CHEMOTHERAPY

- Fertility not affected.

- Immature teratomas can progress rapidly; chemotherapy should be initiated as soon as possible after surgery, preferably within 7-10 days. (N12)

- BEP (bleomycin, etoposide, cisplatin)
  - Bleomycin 30 U/wk, etoposide 100 mg/m^2/d for days 1-5, cisplatin 20 mg/m^2/d for days 1-5
  - Repeat every 21 days for 3 cycles for good risk (category 2B), or 4 cycles for poor risk

- Etoposide/carboplatin (EC)
  - For stage IB-III dysgerminoma for whom minimizing toxicity is critical, 3 courses of etoposide/carboplatin can be used
  - Carboplatin 400 mg/m^2 on day 1 plus etoposide 120 mg/m^2 on days 1, 2, and 3 every 4 weeks for 3 courses.

- Several case reports suggest that patients who have received chemotherapy for germ cell tumors may later present with growing teratoma syndrome.

RADIOTHERAPY (N12)

- Dysgerminomas are **very sensitive to radiation;** doses of 2,500-3,500 cGy may be curative, even for gross metastatis. **Loss of fertility** is a problem with radiation, so rarely used as first-line treatment.

- Not used in immature teratomas also. Reserve it for **localized persistent disease after chemotherapy.**

FOLLOW-UP/MONITORING

- Physical examination every 2-4 months for 2 years f/b every year
- Tumor markers (AFP, β-hCG, LDH) every 2-4 months (if initially elevated) upto 2 years
- Imaging (CXR, CT, MRI) as clinically indicated is done unless markers normal at initial presentation
- If recurrence is suspected CT scan and tumor markers are done during followup.

MANAGEMENT OF RECURRENT DISEASE

- In dysgerminoma ~75% of recurrences occur **within the first year after initial treatment, the most common sites being the peritoneal cavity and the retroperitoneal lymph nodes.**

- High-dose chemotherapy
- Cisplatin/etoposide
- Docetaxel
- Docetaxel/carboplatin
- Paclitaxel
- Paclitaxel/ifosfamide
- Paclitaxel/carboplatin
- Paclitaxel/gemcitabine
- VIP (etoposide, ifosfamide, cisplatin)
- VeIP (vinblastine, ifosfamide, cisplatin)
- VAC (vincristine, dactinomycin, cyclophosphamide)
- TIP (paclitaxel, ifosfamide, cisplatin)
- Radiation therapy (loss of fertility)
- Supportive care only

VAC	
Vincristine	1-1.5 mg/m^2 on day 1 every 4 weeks
Dactinomycin	0.5 mg/day × 5 days every 4 weeks
Cyclophosphamide	150 mg/m^2/day × 5 days every 4 weeks

MANAGEMENT DURING PREGNANCY

- Because dysgerminomas tend to occur in young patients, they may **coexist with pregnancy...**
  - If stage IA, remove the tumor intact and continue the pregnancy.
  - If more advanced disease, continuation of the pregnancy depends on the gestational age of the fetus. **Chemotherapy can be given in the second and third trimesters in the same dosages as given for the nonpregnant patient** without apparent detriment to the fetus. (N12)

LATE EFFECTS OF TREATMENT OF MALIGNANT GERM CELL TUMORS

GONADAL FUNCTION

- Unnecessary BSO and hysterectomy in germ cell tumors can cause infertility.

- Although temporary ovarian dysfunction or failure is common with platinum-based chemotherapy, most women will resume normal ovarian function, and childbearing is usually preserved.

- **Older age at initiation of chemotherapy, greater cumulative drug dose and longer duration of therapy** all have an adverse effect on future gonadal function.

SECONDARY MALIGNANCIES

- An important cause of late morbidity and mortality in patients receiving chemotherapy for germ cell tumors is the development of secondary tumors.

- **Etoposide has been implicated in the development of treatment-related leukemias.**

- The chance of developing **treatment-related leukemia following etoposide** is dose related.

Cumulative etoposide dose	<2,000 mg/m^2	>2,000 mg/m^2
Incidence of leukemia	~0.4-0.5% (30-fold increased likelihood)	5% (336-fold increased likelihood)

- In a typical 3-4 cycle course of BEP, patients receive a cumulative etoposide dose of 1,500 or 2,000 mg/m^2, respectively.

- Despite the risk of secondary leukemia, risk-benefit analyses have concluded that etoposide-containing regimens are beneficial in advanced germ cell tumors; one case of treatment-induced leukemia would be expected for every 20 additionally cured patients who receive BEP as compared with PVB.

SEX CORD STROMAL (5-8%)

INTRODUCTION/EPIDEMIOLOGY

- Account for ~**5-8% of all ovarian Tumors malignancies.**

ORIGIN

- **Derive from the sex cords and the ovarian stroma or mesenchyme.**

- The tumors usually are composed of various combinations of elements, including the **female cells (i.e., granulosa and theca cells) and male cells (i.e., Sertoli and Leydig cells)**, as well as morphologically indifferent cells.

CLASSIFICATION

1. **Granulosa-stromal cell tumors**
    A. Granulosa cell tumor group (adult, juvenile) (MC)
    B. Thecoma-fibroma group
        1. Thecoma
        2. Fibroma
        3. Unclassified (fibrothecoma)
2. **Sertoli-stromal cell tumors**
    A. Androblastomas; Sertoli-Leydig cell tumor group
        1. Well-differentiated
        2. Intermediate differentiation
        3. Poorly differentiated
    B. Sertoli cell tumor
    C. Stromal-Leydig cell tumor
3. **Sex cord stromal tumors of mixed or unclassified cell types**
    A. Gynandroblastoma
    B. Sex cord tumor with annular tubules
    C. Sex cord stromal tumors, unclassified
4. **Steroid cell tumors**
    A. Stromal luteoma
    B. Leydig cell tumor group
        1. Hilus cell tumor
        2. Leydig cell tumor, non-hilar type
        3. Leydig cell tumor, not otherwise specified
    C. Steroid cell tumor, not other classified

GRANULOSA-STROMAL CELL TUMORS

- Include granulosa cell tumors, thecomas and fibromas.

- Low-grade malignancy; rarely, thecomas and fibromas have morphologic features of malignancy and then may be referred to as fibrosarcomas.

- **Bilateral in only 2% of patients.**

- Granulosa cell tumors, which **secrete estrogen**, are **seen in all ages.** Found in prepubertal girls in 5% of cases; the remainders are found in women throughout their reproductive and postmenopausal years...
  - Of the rare prepubertal lesions, 75% have sexual pseudoprecocity,
  - Of reproductive age patients, most have menstrual irregularities or secondary amenorrhea, and cystic hyperplasia of the endometrium is frequently present,
  - Of postmenopausal patients, AUB is frequently the initial symptom. Indeed, the estrogen secretion in them can be sufficient to develop endometrial cancer. **Endometrial cancer occurs in association with granulosa cell tumors in at least 5% of cases,** and 25-50% are associated with endometrial hyperplasia.

- Granulosa tumors tend to be hemorrhagic; occasionally, they **rupture and produce a hemoperitoneum.**

- **Inhibin** is secreted by some granulosa cell tumors. **An elevated serum inhibin level in a premenopausal woman with amenorrhea and infertility is suggestive of a granulosa cell tumor.**

- Malignant thecomas are extremely rare, and their signs and symptoms, management, and outcome is similar to those of the granulosa cell tumors.

PATHOLOGY (N12)

GROSS

- Granulosa cell tumors **range from a few millimeters to 20 centimeters or more** in diameter. The tumors are rarely bilateral, and they have a **smooth, lobulated** surface. The solid portions of the tumor are granular, frequently trabeculated, and are commonly **yellow or gray-yellow** in color.

- After **clear cell carcinoma the granulosa-theca cell tumor is probably the most inaccurately diagnosed** lesion of the female gonad. Lesions misdiagnose as granulosa cell tumors include **metastatic carcinomas, teratoid tumors and poorly differentiated mesothelial tumors.**

MICROSCOPIC

- The classic granulosa cell is **round or ovoid with scant cytoplasm.** The **nucleus contains compact, finely granular chromatin and is either euchromatic or hypochromatic.** "Coffee bean" grooved nuclei are characteristic, mitotic figures may be present, but numerous mitotic figures should prompt consideration for poorly differentiated or undifferentiated carcinoma.

- In the MC variety, the granulosa cells show a tendency to arrange themselves in small clusters or rosettes around a central cavity, so there is a resemblance to primordial follicles (**Call-Exner bodies).**

- The **stroma is similar to the theca** and **may be luteinized.**

- In children and adolescents, the granular cell tumors are often cystic, contain luteinized cells, and can be associated with precocious puberty.

- Juvenile granulosa cell tumors tend to occur in younger patients, feature rounder, more hyperchromatic nuclei and may contain numerous mitotic figures. Large, irregular follicle spaces are additional distinguishing feature of the juvenile granulosa cell tumor.

- The adult granulosa cell tumor tends to occur in older, but the diagnosis is not based on age of presentation, but on histology. Adult granulosa cell tumors, but not juvenile granulosa cell tumors, harbor a somatic mutation in the FOXL2 gene.

PATTERNS OF SPREAD (N12)

- The tumors may also spread hematogenously, and metastases can develop in the lungs, liver, and brain years after initial diagnosis. When adult granulosa cell tumors do recur, they can progress quite rapidly.

PROGNOSIS (N12)

- Most histologic types have the same prognosis, but patients with the more **poorly differentiated diffuse or sarcomatoid type tends to do worse.**

- The **presence of residual disease** is the most important predictor of progression-free survival, but **DNA ploidy** is an independent prognostic factor. Patients with residual-negative DNA diploid tumors had a 10-year PFS of 96%.

- **Adult granulosa cell tumors are usually stage I at diagnosis but may recur 5 to 30 years after initial diagnosis** reflecting their low-grade biology. **10-year survival rate is** ~**90%, with 20-year survival rates dropping to 75%.**

- Juvenile granulosa cell tumors are...
- Rare,
- Mostly clinically benign & 10% are malignant,
- Make up less than 5% of ovarian tumors in childhood and adolescence,
- 90% are diagnosed in stage I,
- Having favorable prognosis,
- Less aggressive than adult type,
- Only ~10% recur and when they do so, it is generally within 5 years of the initial diagnosis.

SERTOLI-LEYDIG TUMORS

- Most frequently in the **3rd and 4th decades; 75% are seen in women <40 yrs.**

- Extremely rare and account for **less than 0.2% of ovarian cancers.**

- Most frequently **low-grade malignancies,** although occasionally **a poorly differentiated variety may behave more aggressively.**

- The tumors typically **produce androgens,** and clinical virilization is noted in 70-85% of patients. Measurement of plasma androgens may reveal elevated testosterone and androstenedione, with normal or slightly elevated DHEA-S.

- Rarely, the Sertoli-Leydig tumor can be associated with **manifestations of estrogenization** (i.e., isosexual precocity, irregular, or postmenopausal bleeding).

- Rarely bilateral (<1%).

PROGNOSIS (N12)

- The 5-year survival rate is 70-90% and recurrences thereafter are uncommon. Most fatalities occur in the presence of poorly differentiated lesions.

MANAGEMENT OF MALIGNANT SEX CORD STROMAL TUMORS

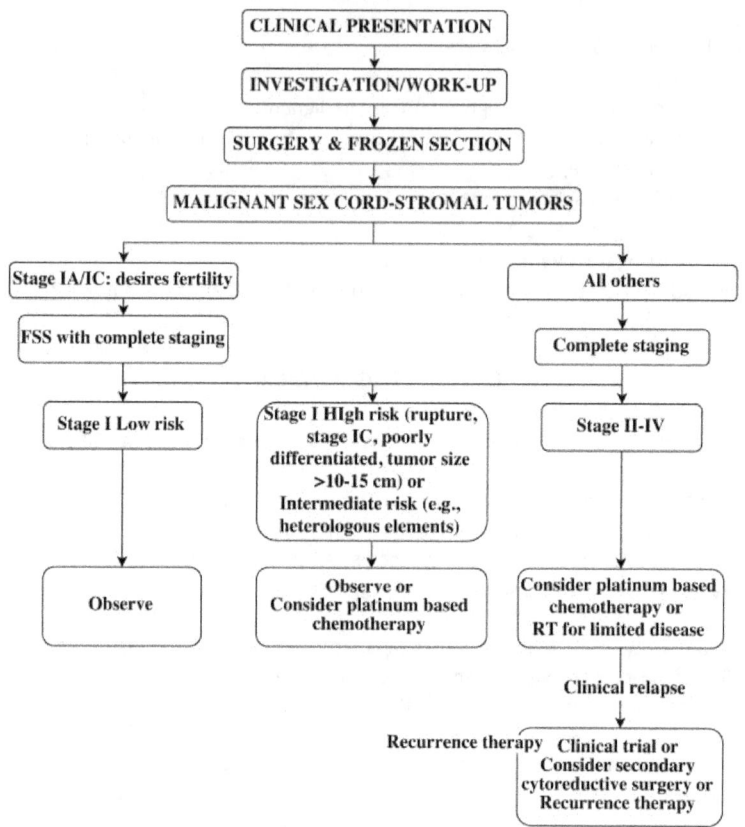

PRIMARY TREATMENT

SURGICAL STAGING FOR EARLY STAGE & PRIMARY CYTOREDUCTIVE SURGERY FOR ADVANCED STAGE

- Basic principles already mentioned.

- Although complete staging is recommended for all who doesn't desire fertility, lymphadenectomy may be omitted.

- FSS for those desiring fertility & should be monitored by ultrasound if necessary; completion surgery (category 2B) after finishing childbearing.

POST OPERATIVE CHEMOTHERAPY/PRIMARY CHEMOTHERAPY/ADJUVANT CHEMOTHERAPY

- BEP or paclitaxel/carboplatin regimens.

FOLLOW-UP/MONITORING

- Prolonged surveillance is recommended for granulosa cell tumors, because they can recur years later.

- Physical examination every 2-4 months for 2 years f/b **every 6 months**
- Tumor markers (inhibin) every 2-4 months (if initially elevated) upto 2 years **f/b every 6 months**
- Imaging (CXR, CT, MRI) **insufficient data to show role**
- If recurrence is suspected CT scan and tumor markers are done during followup.

MANAGEMENT OF RECURRENT DISEASE

- Granulosa cell tumors are potentially hormonally responsive, with about 30% of granulosa tumors expressing estrogen receptors and almost 100% expressing progesterone receptors. Hormonal agents, such as **progestins or LHRH agonists** are used to treat because they are often elderly. There are case reports of durable response to **aromatase inhibitors** in patients with metastatic granulosa cell tumors who received multiple prior treatment.

- Secondary cytoreductive surgery
- Aromatase inhibitors (anastrozole, letrozole)
- Bevacizumab may be considered for **granulosa cell tumors**
- Leuprolide may be used as hormonal therapy for **granulosa cell tumors**
- Docetaxel
- Paclitaxel
- Paclitaxel/ifosfamide
- Paclitaxel/carboplatin
- Tamoxifen
- VAC
- Radiation therapy
- Supportive care only

UNCOMMON OVARIAN CANCERS

- Only 0.1% of all ovarian malignancies.

LIPOID CELL TUMORS

- **Arise in adrenal cortical rests** that **reside in the vicinity of the ovary.**

- Bilateral disease has been noted in only a few.

- Associated with virilization, obesity, hypertension, and glucose intolerance reflecting corticosteroid secretion. Rare cases of estrogen secretion and isosexual precocity have been reported.

- Have benign or low-grade behavior, but about 20%, most of which are initially >8 cm in diameter, are associated with metastatic lesions in the peritoneal cavity.

- The primary treatment is surgical extirpation of the primary lesion. There are no data regarding the effectiveness of radiation or chemotherapy for this disease.

SARCOMAS/CARCINOSARCOMAS/ MALIGNANT MIXED MESODERMAL TUMORS (MMMT)

- Monoclonal & are metaplastic carcinomas in which the mesenchymal part reflects dedifferentiation.

- A variant of poor risk, poorly differentiated EOC (metaplastic carcinoma).

- Most lesions are **heterologous**, and **80% occur in postmenopausal women.** Biologically aggressive, having poor prognosis and most have **evidence of metastases** at presentation.

MANAGEMENT

- NO FSS regardless of age.
- Optimal surgical debulking is recommended.
- After complete surgical staging, all should have postoperative chemotherapy.

- Patients with stage I to IV MMMT or recurrence are treated using the same chemotherapy regimens that are recommended for EOC.

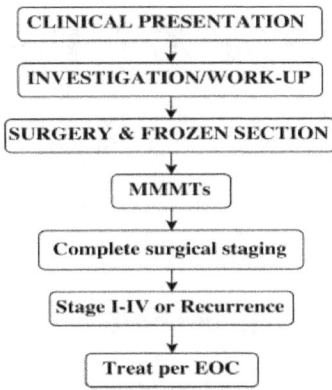

```
┌─────────────────────────────┐
│   CLINICAL PRESENTATION      │
└─────────────────────────────┘
              ↓
┌─────────────────────────────┐
│   INVESTIGATION/WORK-UP      │
└─────────────────────────────┘
              ↓
┌─────────────────────────────┐
│  SURGERY & FROZEN SECTION    │
└─────────────────────────────┘
              ↓
      ┌───────────────┐
      │    MMMTs       │
      └───────────────┘
              ↓
   ┌────────────────────────┐
   │ Complete surgical staging│
   └────────────────────────┘
              ↓
    ┌──────────────────────┐
    │ Stage I-IV or Recurrence│
    └──────────────────────┘
              ↓
       ┌───────────────┐
       │  Treat per EOC │
       └───────────────┘
```

SMALL CELL CARCINOMAS

- This rare tumor occurs at an average age of 24 yr (range 2-46 years).

- The tumors are typically unilateral.

- 2/3rd of the tumors are accompanied by paraendocrine hypercalcemia. This tumor accounts for **one half of all of the cases of hypercalcemia associated with ovarian tumors.**

- ~50% of the tumors have spread beyond the ovaries when they are diagnosed.

- Immunohistochemical stains are helpful to differentiate this tumor from a lymphoma, leukemia or sarcoma.

- Management consists of **surgery followed by platinum-based chemotherapy or radiation therapy or both.** In addition to the primary treatment of the disease, control of the **hypercalcemia may require aggressive hydration, loop diuretics, and the use of bisphosphonates or calcitonin.**

- The prognosis tends to be poor, with most dying within 2 years of diagnosis in spite of treatment.

METASTATIC TUMORS

- ~5-6% of ovarian tumors are metastatic from other organs, most frequently from the female genital tract, the breast, or the GI tract.

- Metastases may occur from direct extension of another pelvic neoplasm, by hematogenous or lymphatic spread, or by transcoelomic dissemination, with surface implantation of tumors that spread in the peritoneal cavity.

GYNECOLOGIC

- Non-ovarian cancers of the genital tract can spread by direct extension or they may metastasize to the ovaries.

- **Tubal carcinoma** involves the ovaries secondarily in 13% of cases, usually by direct extension. Under some circumstances, it is difficult to know whether the tumor originated in the tube or in the ovary when both are involved.

- **Cervical cancer** spreads to the ovary only in rare cases (<1%), and most of these are of an advanced clinical stage or are adenocarcinomas.

- Although **adenocarcinoma of the endometrium** can spread and implant directly onto the surface of the ovaries in as many as 5% of cases, two synchronous primary tumors probably occur with greater frequency. In these cases, an **endometrioid carcinoma of the ovary is usually associated with the adenocarcinoma of the endometrium.**

NONGYNECOLOGIC

BREAST CARCINOMA

- In autopsy data of women who died of metastatic breast cancer, the ovaries were involved in 24% of cases, and 80% of the involvement was bilateral. Similarly, when ovaries are removed to palliate advanced breast cancer, about 20-30% of the cases reveal ovarian involvement, 60% of those bilaterally.

- The involvement of ovaries in early-stage breast cancer seems to be considerably lower. In almost all cases, either ovarian involvement is occult or a pelvic mass is discovered after other metastatic disease becomes apparent.

KRUKENBERG TUMOR

- The Krukenberg tumor, which can account for **30-40% of metastatic cancers** to the ovaries, arises in the ovarian stroma and has **characteristic mucin-filled, signet-ring cells.**

- The primary tumor is most frequently located in the stomach and less commonly in the colon, appendix (so called- goblet cell carcinoid), breast, or biliary tract. Rarely, the cervix or the bladder may be the primary site.

- Krukenberg tumors can account for ~2% of ovarian cancers, and are usually **bilateral.** The lesions are usually not discovered until the primary disease is advanced and, therefore, most patients die of their disease within 1 year. In some cases, a primary tumor is never found.

OTHER GASTROINTESTINAL TUMORS

- In other cases of metastasis from the gastrointestinal tract to the ovary, the tumor does not have the classic histologic appearance of a Krukenberg tumor; most of these are from the colon and, less commonly, the pancreato-billiary tract, appendix and the small intestine.

- As many as **1-2% of women with intestinal carcinomas will develop metastases to the ovaries** during the course of their disease.

- Before exploration for an adnexal tumor in a **woman older than 40 years, a barium enema is indicated** to exclude a primary gastrointestinal carcinoma with metastases to the ovaries, **particularly if there are any gastrointestinal symptoms.**

- Metastatic colon cancer can **mimic a mucinous cystadenocarcinoma of the ovary** histologically and the histological distinction between the two can be difficult. Lesions that arise in the appendix may be associated with ovarian metastasis and have frequently been confused with primary ovarian malignancies, especially when associated with pseudomyxoma peritonei. Therefore, it is reasonable to consider the performance of prophylactic BSO at the time of surgery for women with colon cancer.

MELANOMA

- Rare cases of malignant melanoma metastatic to the ovaries have been reported.

- In these circumstances, the melanomas are usually widely disseminated. Removal would be warranted for palliation of abdominal or pelvic pain, bleeding, or torsion.

- Malignant melanoma can arise rarely in a mature cystic teratoma.

CARCINOID TUMORS

- Metastatic carcinoid tumors represent **fewer than 2% of metastatic lesions to the ovaries.**

- Conversely, **only about 2% of patients with primary carcinoids have evidence of ovarian metastasis**, and only 40% of them have the carcinoid syndrome at the time of discovery of the metastatic carcinoid.

- However, in perimenopausal and postmenopausal women explored for an intestinal carcinoid, it is reasonable to remove the ovaries to prevent subsequent ovarian metastasis. Furthermore, the discovery of an ovarian carcinoid should prompt a careful search for a primary intestinal lesion.

LYMPHOMA AND LEUKEMIA

- Lymphomas and leukemia can involve the ovary. When they do, the involvement is **usually bilateral.**

- About **5% of patients with Hodgkin disease** will have lymphomatous involvement of the ovaries, but this involvement occurs typically with advanced-stage disease.

- With **Burkitt's lymphoma**, ovarian involvement is very common.

- Other types of lymphoma involve the **ovaries much less frequently,** and leukemic infiltration of the ovaries is uncommon.

- Sometimes the ovaries can be the only apparent site of involvement of the abdominal or pelvic viscera with a lymphoma; if this circumstance is found, a careful surgical exploration may be necessary. Intraoperatively, a hematologist-oncologist should be consulted to determine the need for these procedures if frozen section of a solid ovarian mass reveals a lymphoma. In general, most lymphomas no longer require extensive surgical staging, although biopsy of enlarged lymph nodes should generally be performed. In some cases of Hodgkin disease, a more extensive evaluation may be necessary. Treatment involves that of the lymphoma or leukemia in general. Removal of a large ovarian mass may improve patient comfort and facilitate a response to subsequent radiation or chemotherapy.

MISCELLANEOUS

ROLE OF LAPAROSCOPY IN THE MANAGEMENT OF OVARIAN CANCER

- Open laparotomy should be used for patients with suspected malignant ovarian cancer if the treatment plan involves surgical staging, primary debulking, interval debulking, or secondary cytoreduction. if patients cannot be optimally debulked using minimally invasive techniques, they should be converted to an open procedure. (N15)

(a) Primary surgery for early-stage ovarian cancer (most useful),
(b) Restaging of unstaged ovarian cancer (most useful),
(c) Primary cytoreductive surgery for advanced-stage ovarian cancer,
(d) Assessment of resectability (most useful) in patients with advanced-stage disease to determine whether primary cytoreductive surgery or neoadjuvant chemotherapy and interval debulking is preferable [Currently, a prospective randomized trial is being conducted in Europe where patients with advanced ovarian cancer (stage IIIC) will undergo laparoscopic assessment of tumor volume and then proceed with an attempt at cytoreduction versus neoadjuvant chemotherapy. This trial is known as the SCORPION trial (Surgical Complications Related to Primary or Interval Debulking in Ovarian Neoplasm)],
(e) Intraperitoneal catheter placement,
(f) Second-look surgery, and
(g) Secondary cytoreductive surgery. (T15)

- The major concern regarding the use of laparoscopic surgery in the management of ovarian cancer is spread of the cancer, particularly port site metastasis (1-2%).

FERTILITY SPARING SURGERY (FSS)

AIM:

- To preserve reproductive potential without compromising curability.

PRINCIPLE:

- If cancer is confined to one ovary → USO.
- If mass is benign → ovarian cystectomy. The specimen should be sent for frozen section. If malignancy is diagnosed, then appropriate staging biopsies should be performed.

- If C/L ovary appears normal, it should not be biopsied to avoid potential infertility caused by peritoneal adhesions or ovarian failure.

CRITERIA:

- Patient desirous of preserving fertility.
- Patient and family consent and agree to close follow-up.
- **No evidence of dysgenetic gonads.**
- Specific situations:
  - Any unilateral malignant germ-cell tumor.
  - Any unilateral sex cord stromal tumor (IA, IC).
  - Stage IA, IC invasive epithelial tumor.
  - Any unilateral borderline tumor.

MALIGNANT GERM CELL TUMORS:

- 50% to 70% of malignant germ-cell tumors are stage I.
- Except for dysgerminoma, in which the incidence of bilaterality is 10-15%, bilateral ovarian tumors are rare.
- Benign cystic teratoma is associated with malignant germ-cell tumors in 5-10% of cases and may occur in one or both ovaries.

- USO + surgical staging is performed in these neoplasms, even many with advanced-stage disease.
- If C/L ovary is enlarged, mostly it represents a benign cystic teratoma → ovarian cystectomy.
- Postop chemoRx of BEP regime is required (mainly for serum tumor marker elevation) in malignant germ cell tumors except...
  - Stage I pure dysgerminoma,
  - Stage I grade 1 immature teratoma.

SEX CORD STROMAL TUMORS:

- Mostly confined to the ovary.
- >50% of granulosa cell tumors → stage I.
- >90% of sertoli-leydig cell tumors → stage IA.
- Bilaterality of granulosa cell & sertoli-leydig cell tumors → <5%.

- USO + surgical staging + endometrial biopsy or curettage (in young patient as 5-15% of patients with granulosa cell tumors develop endometrial cancer or hyperplasia).
- Postop chemoRx of BEP regime or paclitaxel + carboplatin combination is required in...
  - Stage II-IV, and

- o   Stage I high risk (e.g., rupture, IC, poorly differentiated, tumor size >10-15 cm) or intermediate risk (heterologus elements).

INVASIVE EPITHELIAL TUMORS:

- 90% of all ovarian malignancies → Invasive epithelial tumors.
- Despite the low overall survival rate associated with these tumors, selected young patients with stage I disease (Stage IA, IC all grades) can be treated conservatively.
- Conservative Rx depends on...
  - o   Stage,
  - o   Histologic grade, and
  - o   Bilaterality (50% of serous tumors, 5-20% of mucinous tumors, 30-50% of endometrioid and clear-cell cancers are bilateral).

BORDERLINE OR LOW MALIGNANT POTENTIAL OVARIAN TUMORS:

- 10-15% of all ovarian neoplasms are of the borderline or low malignant potential.
- 33-60% of serous borderline tumors are → stage IA. Extraovarian spread is seen in →20-30% of cases.
- 80-90% of mucinous borderline tumors are → stage IA.
- Most of endometrioid and clear-cell borderline tumors are → stage IA.

- If tumor is confined to one ovary...
  - o   USO + surgical staging, or
  - o   Ovarian cystectomy with risk of repeat surgery for a recurrence of tumor in the same or opposite ovary.
- If tumor is bilateral...
  - o   B/L ovarian cystectomy.

- 5-year survival rates with stage I borderline tumors treated with surgery alone → ≥95%.

- If peritoneal implants are present in borderline tumors surgical excision is the mainstay of treatment f/b resection of all gross disease, cytologic washing and staging biopsies of peritoneal surfaces and lymph nodes.
The relapse risk for patients with peritoneal implants is related to the type...
  - o   In noninvasive peritoneal implants, the LR is → 20%.
  - o   In invasive peritoneal implants, the LR is → 50%. Consequently, postoperative platinum-based chemotherapy is recommended (benefit not proved).

IN PRESENT ERA:

- Though women underwent BSO, donor oocyte transfer and hormonal support allows her to sustain a normal intrauterine pregnancy.
- If TAH + USO is done because of tumor involvement, current techniques allow retrieval of oocytes from the patient's remaining ovary, in vitro fertilization with sperm from her male partner, and implantation of the embryo into a surrogate's uterus.

INTESTINAL OBSTRUCTION

INCIDENCE

- ~25% of ovarian cancer patients develop intestinal obstruction in the terminal phase of their illness

- Patients with epithelial ovarian cancer often develop intestinal obstruction, either at the time of initial diagnosis or, more frequently, in association with recurrent disease. Obstruction may be related to a mechanical blockage or to carcinomatous ileus.

CAUSE

- Adhesions; particularly if abdominopelvic radiotherapy is given,
- Progressive tumor.

SITE

- The site(s) may be solitary or multiple...
  - Simultaneous obstruction of the small and large bowel (5-10%).
  - Colon obstruction (33%) usually occurs in the area of the sigmoid colon because of growth of pelvic tumor and resultant extrinsic compression; occasionally there may be obstruction of more proximal segments.
  - Small bowel obstruction (50%) is usually the result of adherence of loops of bowel by mesenteric or serosal tumor implants.

CLINICAL FEATURES

- Nausea, vomiting, abdominal cramping, abdominal distention, and progressive constipation.
- In partial obstruction, these symptoms may be episodic and more subtle.

DIAGNOSIS

- Routine abdominal X-ray shows...
  - Dilatation of the small intestine and air fluid levels (small bowel obstruction),
  - Dilatation of the colon (large bowel obstruction),
  - Nonspecific findings (early & partial obstruction).

- CT abdomen pelvis provides information regarding sites of obstruction & degree of carcinomatosis.

TREATMENT

- Can be corrected if obstruction **appears at the time of initial diagnosis.**
  - If life expectancy is very short (e.g., <2 months), presence of bulky carcinomatosis, rapidly progressive disease, multiple sites of obstruction, poor performance status, or heavy pretreatment with chemotherapy and radiation; surgical relief is not indicated.
  - If life span is longer, features that predict a reasonable likelihood of correcting the obstruction include **young age, good nutritional status & the absence of rapidly accumulating ascites.**

- Optimal **preoperative preparation** is desirable if a patient is judged to be a suitable candidate for surgical intervention.
  - Proper radiographic documentation of the obstruction,
  - Hydration,
  - Correction of any electrolyte disturbances,
  - Parenteral alimentation (in malnourished, places patient in an anabolic state & decreases postoperative morbidity),
  - Intestinal intubation,
  - Antibiotics.

For some, the obstruction may be alleviated by this conservative approach.

- **For patients with complete colonic obstruction or perforation of the small or large intestine,** a surgical emergency exists unless the patient is in such poor condition that such an intervention is not feasible. **Colonic obstruction** usually is treated by performing a colostomy. The selection of the site of colostomy depends on the area of obstruction and the ability to find an adequate bowel segment free of cancer. Most commonly, a transverse loop colostomy is indicated in the presence of a descending colon or sigmoid colon obstruction. There is increasing experience with the use of colonic stents as a substitute for colostomy. Patient selection is key, because erosion of the colonic wall with perforation is a risk.

- Emergency surgery is rarely indicated in small intestinal obstruction. It is preferable to optimize the patient's condition with nasogastric tube decompression and rehydration. In addition, a barium enema is usually indicated to rule out a coexisting colonic obstruction. Management for **small bowel obstruction** depends on the operative findings.

- Multiple sites of obstruction in the terminal ileum → ileo-ascending colon bypass, ileo-transverse colon bypass. Resection and reanastomosis are inappropriate.
- An isolated area of obstruction → Resection and reanastomosis (either hand sewn using a two-layer technique or approximated with surgical staplers).
- Extensive tumor with multiple areas of obstruction → Bypass and resection impossible. A tube gastrostomy is indicated in such a situation, if possible. Enterotomies are not uncommon and should be repaired as soon as they are identified.

Complications of small intestinal procedures include wound infection, intraperitoneal abscess, sepsis, pneumonia, blind loop syndrome and enterocutaneous fistula.

PROGNOSIS

- **Surgery carries an operative mortality of ~10% and a major complications rate of about 30%.** The need for multiple reanastomoses and prior radiation therapy increase the morbidity, which consists primarily of sepsis and enterocutaneous fistulae. The median survival ranges from 3-12 months, although about 20% of such patients survive longer than 12 months.

Thank you...

:FURTHER READING:

Berek & Noak's Gynecology, 14, 15th edition (N12)
Te Linde's OPERATIVE GYNECOLOGY, 10, 11th edition (T15)
FIGO's staging classification for cancer of the ovary, fallopian tube, and peritoneum: JGO 2015
NCCN guidelines for management of ovarian cancer 2015 (N15)
Green top guidelines (R11, R10)